Hope I Dont Die
Before I Get Old

DEDICATION

We dedicate this book to every child, friend, parent, relation and professional who set aside their own interests to help another in their time of need. You are the real life heroes. In small kindnesses, true greatness is revealed.

"There are only four kinds of people in the world:
Those who have been caretakers,
Those who currently are caretakers,
Those who will be caretakers,
And those who will need caretakers."

Rosalynn Carter

"Age is an issue of mind over matter. If you don't mind, it doesn't matter."

Mark Twain

they lived on beyond their independence—we suffered from it, too. In fact, as Boomers we were probably even less prepared than our parents, for they at least believed in the post-WWII concept of saving for the future. We hadn't been able to save very much for our retirement, mostly because we had been too busy taking care of our kids, our careers, not to mention our parents.

As we looked ahead, aghast, we saw that time was running out and that we had no actual, reliable plan in place for our own aging journey. Just like our parents! We yelped a collective, "Yikes! We have to do something about this!" We decided we had to find a path through the thickets of denial and false hope. We needed to discover a new way to tackle our inevitable old age. We had learned a lot about how not to age from taking care of our parents. We had seen firsthand how awful it was to ignore very real limitations and, in doing so, forgo any hope for healing, or support. We sought to understand more about this process and to change our point of view so we might go into our older years with more serenity, less panic.

This book is not about denying the reality of aging. We tell our stories of caregiving as homage to our parents' struggles and as cautionary tales for the would-be caregivers out there who, like us, find themselves in strange and unfamiliar territory, looking for a GPS signal.

We tell these stories because in doing so we hope to avoid the same mistakes as we move inexorably into old age, (or so we hope—for old age certainly "beats the alternative," as Maurice Chevalier said.)

Here is one of the biggest things we learned: you need a plan. One of the biggest mistakes one could make is not to have a plan in place. A plan will make it possible to live the best life you can at any age. If you have a plan, you can focus on actually living the kind of life you want, instead of passively waiting for your life to wind down and letting others make your choices for you by default. A plan for your old age is a great gift to your children or would-be caretakers.

As Tracey says, "The goal is to keep being energized by living, to keep growing mentally and spiritually, and to keep as active as possible. You need a plan so that can happen. For anyone to feel that their best years are behind them and that they have nothing to offer or add or create has got to be profoundly depressing."

Our goal for ourselves is to turn our own aging into an extreme sport. In this sport, we can train, we can play, and we can win. We, the authors, are not old. Not yet. We are pre-old. We are in our fifties and sixties and approaching the first blushing youth of our old age, what journalists coyly call "the young old."

Because we are alive now and not a hundred or even fifty years ago, we are already benefiting from better health and ever more amazing medical advances. No surprise, the fastest growing demographic is now people over age eighty-five. They are known as "the old old."

Given our health and education, chances are we are more likely than our parents to keep busy and well. In fact, most boomers will continue to work long past the old traditional retirement age of sixty-five. Many of us will rack up multiple careers, layering up double and triple retirement funds. We may grow old, but many of us will stay fully engaged in our lives. Our generation will be writing a new paradigm for aging.

But before a new paradigm can take off, we thought it a good idea to first understand the state of aging now. How did we get to this particular junction in the road? The stories we share about our parents serve as mile markers. Once we know where we are coming from, going forward in the right direction is going to be a lot easier. Our goal is to take the aging journey to a whole new level. So join us. Let's create the old age we want instead of the one we fear.

CHAPTER TWO
The First Signs of Trouble:
A Visit to the Emergency Room

Tracey

takes a phone call

that ushers in twenty years of slow decline.

Nothing ever really prepares you for that call where you learn that your elderly mother or father is in real trouble. My mother had been ill off and on for much of my life, so I was used to her medical problems by this time. When Mary called from her mom's house, I could hear the anxiety and fear in her voice. But I could also hear the frustration and downright anger at this sudden turn of events. I knew exactly how she felt. I knew how it felt when suddenly, through no fault of your own, you have to drop everything to take care of your parent.

I was used to being called into the "fix-it" mode and yet thinking back I can remember that one phone call that stands out, that ushered in what I call "the beginning" of my mom becoming old. I can easily recall my sister's frantic voice on the phone saying: "Tracey, Mom is in so much pain, lying in bed with her legs curled up, moaning. Mom thought she was just sick feeling from eating too much on Thanksgiving, but it has been two days now and it is getting worse."

My sister didn't know what to do, except to call me because I am "the nurse" as I am often referred to in my family, as if I have all the answers! Mom had driven up from her little apartment in Rhode Island to spend Thanksgiving with us—her two daughters (my sister and I lived near each other in southern New Hampshire). Mom seemed fine at dinner. At age sixty-five, she was her usual self, sharing the meal and her stories with her grandchildren. I listened incredulously as I heard my sister say, "She says her back hurts and her stomach hurts and all she can do is moan!" As a nurse and midwife, I knew it meant something was really wrong, either kidneys, bladder or intestines; a blockage, an infection?

It was seven o'clock, Sunday night, and I was on call and would have to go to the hospital at some point to see a patient who was in the beginning stages of labor. I glanced at my watch, looking at my family eating our dinner, thinking about getting the kids to bed before I got called away and now annoyed to add another responsibility to my load. How do I have time to go see Mom as well? was running through my head as I listened to my sister. It was snowing hard and my sister was alone with her two young daughters. "The pain is getting worse and I don't know what to do," my sister said. "I can't stand this anymore!" This seemed serious. "Take her to the hospital!" I said, while she responded with, "I can't leave the girls alone!" With much sighing and moaning on my part, I said, "Okay, I will come over and look at her before I go to the hospital."

When I got to my sister's house, Mom was huddled in a ball in my sister's bed, heaped with warm blankets, rocking and moaning. As I examined my mom, I quickly realized that she was having kidney and bladder pain. Why? The cause could have been an infection, kidney stones, or even appendicitis. She needed further evaluation and testing. I told mom, "You need to go to the hospital." She just moaned in agreement.

A lot of our elders are coping with at least one of the following conditions, and many are dealing with two or more of the following:

- Heart conditions (hypertension, vascular disease, congestive heart failure, high blood pressure, and coronary artery disease)
- Dementia, including Alzheimer's disease
- Depression
- Incontinence (urine and stool)
- Arthritis
- Osteoporosis
- Diabetes
- Breathing problems
- Frequent falls, which can lead to fractures
- Parkinson's disease
- Cancer
- Eye problems (cataracts, glaucoma, macular degeneration)

As the body ages, changes to be aware of are:

- A slowed reaction time, which is especially important when judging if a person can drive.
- Thinner skin, which can lead to breakdowns and wounds that don't heal quickly.
- A weakened immune system, which can make fighting off viruses, bacteria, and diseases difficult.
- Diminished sense of taste or smell, especially for smokers, which can lead to diminished appetite and diminished awareness of thirst, which can lead to malnutrition and dehydration.

Coronary Artery Disease

Otherwise known as heart disease or cardiovascular disease, CAD may present suddenly with dramatic symptoms. Sometimes there is a gradual onset of signs and symptoms of minor heart problems and are commonly called angina, mild heart attacks, or 'a weak heart.' Artherosclerosis is a major cause of heart disease because it is a build up of plaque in the walls of the arteries which makes it more difficult for blood to flow carrying oxygen to your heart.

Risk Factors:
- Smoking
- Obesity
- High blood pressure
- Age (men over age 45, women over age 55)
- Diabetes

Symptoms:
- Chest pain that is severe, unexpected, and occurs with shortness of breath, sweating, nausea, or weakness.
- Fast heart rate, more than 150 beats per minute.
- Shortness of breath not relieved by rest.
- Sudden weakness or paralysis in the arms or legs.
- Sudden, severe headache.
- Fatigue
- Fainting spell with loss of consciousness.

For a helpful tool to create your own heart health program go to:
http://mylifecheck.heart.org/
www.heart.org
http://www.ncbi.nlm.nih.gov/pubmedhealth/PMH0004449/

CHAPTER THREE
Recovery at a Snail's Pace

Mary Boone

drives from New Hampshire to Virginia

and

back again, and back again, and back again,

stopping only for a kiss for Mom, and feeding the cats

or possibly kissing the cats and feeding Mom—it gets to be a blur after

7,952 miles.

If the journey with my mother began with a phone call, then I really should not have been surprised at how walking the journey with her would require umpteen million calls: calls to find information, calls to locate agencies that provided services for the elderly; calls to locate handrails for her bathroom, and calls to order a variety of nutritious and delicious, easy-to-prepare meals for when I was gone. Most of all, there were the calls to my brother to keep him up to date on Mom's progress. I quickly learned not to waste time sharing my frustrations with my brother; I just gave him the rather undramatic bulletins. He was already upset; no need to stir that pot. Instead, I called Tracey for emotional support.

During those first days, I rallied my natural "can-do" resources. I was lucky. I had the time, money, and energy to help. I was not caught between taking care of my family and taking care of my mother or my job. My children were all grown. My business could function without my physical presence. I lived alone in a well-maintained house while my daughter and friends took care of the cats. Good timing, Mom—this was the first time in my life I had few formal claims on my time and was free to help. After all, I thought, Mom cared for me and gave me everything I needed for eighteen years and this was the least I could do. I vowed to stay as long as I was needed and to make Mom's last years happy, even if it killed me.

And so I cooked, I cleaned, I did laundry, all the while my mother simmered with aggravation at having someone in her house, even if that someone was her very own daughter. Then again, she was coping with her first real health crisis that was not a crisis, but rather a symptom of what we both could not yet talk about: her aging and her need for help.

The sight of my mother "failing" had me in the grip of a panic and turned me into a whiny sniveling complainer to Tracey and my other friends I called with updates. I realized that as long as I was talking about how bad I felt, I had no time to consider what was behind my pain and anger. One friend even pointed out that at least I had a mother to complain about. (I had tactlessly included her in my daily festival of cranky emails, forgetting that she had nursed both her parents through their last illnesses years before.)

Each time I saw Mom struggle to keep her balance or try to eat the nice meals I put in front of her, for which she clearly had no appetite, I worried that this was, indeed, the beginning of the end. I was not ready to lose my mother. Nor was I ready to see the path of her decline ahead, so up close and personal; a path I would be faced with sooner or later for myself. Watching her struggle, I could not help but realize, in time, no matter how much I exercised, ate power foods in the right combination, sought out weird or ancient therapies to preserve my youthful vigor, no

Raised Toilet Seat

This is a nifty device that will make getting up and down from the toilet much safer and easier on unsteady legs. It can be installed in a few minutes with simple tools.

Big Number Phones

If vision is an issue, or when glasses are misplaced, get a phone with an oversized keypad. This is an easy fix for better communication. Some have speed dial buttons which can be customized with photos.

Amplified Phones

These come with a broader range of volume control and are good for those with hearing loss.

Lighting

This is one of the easiest things to fix. Replace dark lamp shades with light ones and swap the bulbs for ones with higher wattages. Dimmer switches and three-way bulbs are also a help so you can get higher light levels when needed and a more relaxing atmosphere when not.

Night lights are important to ensure safe passage between rooms, and you can get ones with motion and light detectors built in so it is not necessary to turn them on and off. A few styles come with their own battery back in case of power outage. Some can be used as a flashlight, too.

Grabber Tongs

These are nifty long handled tongs that pick items off the floor or a high shelf. They help prevent accidents when reaching down or up for an elusive object.

Daily Medication Boxes

To ensure proper dosage and compliance, these are handy little boxes with the days of the week and multiple dose compartments so you can see at a glance if a medication has been skipped. There are now medicine-dispensing boxes that hold a week's worth of medicine that sound an alert when it is time to take the dose. You can find these at: www.epill.com.

A Good Cane

Canes should be adjusted to the proper height for the user. Consider a rolling cart, which doubles as a seat and carrying device. My mom's has a cup holder and compartment under the seat for purse, sweater, etc.

The Internet

Web access has been a great boon to people who don't get out as much as they used to. A small laptop is inexpensive, relatively easy to master, and will open up a world of entertainment and information options for the elderly. It is a fun way to bring the generations together, so consider asking a great niece or nephew to be on hand for tech support.

GPS Tracking Devices

If your loved one tends to wander off. Using a phone with GPS tracking is another easy way to keep track of them. There are watch-like GPS devices available for this purpose as well, which have the advantage of being attached to a wrist.

Portable Scooters

These are a great idea if mobility is an issue and limits what adventures can be taken on. These fit into most cars and could make it possible to take grandma along on an outing she otherwise would not have the stamina for. These scooters are very heavy, so be sure you have a ramp and vehicle that one accommodate the scooter. Note: Save these scooters for special outings and don't make it too easy for everyday short-trip use. This way you do not lose valuable exercise opportunities.

In addition to Costco, www.costco.com, for a fun shopping expedition, go to these websites to see the latest gadgets for home safety:

http://www.seniorssuperstores.com

http://www.activeforever.com

Mary Boone's Guide to Opening the Door to Your Helpers

- If you live long enough, you are probably going to need help.

- People who love you get a lot of satisfaction from lending a hand.

- Be generous and let them help you, so you can keep building on your relationships right up until you leave (euphemism for die.)

- Get paid helpers for long-term needs or after surgery days, so your friends and relatives can offer what they can without guilt over the fact that you need more than they can give.

- Have a plan in case you have unexpected needs. No one plans to fall, have a stroke, or be in a car accident. If you are taken by surprise, wouldn't it be great for everyone if you spelled out how you would like to be cared for, rather than making others figure it out?

- If you get anxious around surgeries, appointments or other things that are scheduled, get help for that before you get all crabby and drive your loved ones away. A deep breath is a start.

- Express your appreciation—tell people how much their support means to you.

- Finally, have a few copies of the serenity prayer around, for yourself and your helpers.

God grant me the serenity
to accept the things I cannot change;
courage to change the things I can;
and wisdom to know the difference.

Reinhold Niebuhr

Even though this prayer is the one used in AA, I recommend a glass of wine all around to ease the tensions and burdens on both sides of the care equation, provided you have no problem with alcohol.

If it is beyond your capacity to take comfort from this, then google the TV episode "Serenity Now, Seinfeld" and check out the YouTube clip of this famous episode. Sit back and be prepared to have TV give you a look in the mirror; I guarantee it will lighten your mood!

"The great secret that all old people share is that you really haven't changed in seventy or eighty years. Your body changes, but you don't change at all. And that, of course, causes great confusion."

Doris Lessing

Mom, to see how things were going so I would know when action was truly needed. I had learned the hard way that Mom was all too adept at "spinning" her story to keep my brother and me from worrying, even while she was afraid her strength would fail her. I asked around and found an independent geriatric registered nurse who would make home visits.

Louise Mohardt is a qualified geriatric nurse practitioner, BSRN, who has an independent practice as a geriatric care manager in the region. Geriatric care managers are often former nurses or social workers who have gone on to become certified in geriatric care management. The certification is important because it sets a standard of skills and responsibility which ensures you are getting the very best advice and support, wherever you are in the country. The agency that does these certifications is the National Association of Professional Geriatric Care Managers (NAPGCM). This certified professional is a vital expert to have on your team. You can find out more about care managers and a list of them in your area at their website: www.caremanager.org.

After Louise came for an in-home consultation, I was hopeful she would be a big help in keeping Mom's health on track. Louise was mature, accomplished, and tactful. Best of all, she had a great sense of humor and could lighten up even the most unpalatable topics, from managing toilet issues to determining whether driving is still safe for an elderly person. My mother and I took a liking to Louise right away. Most geriatric care managers charge by the hour, about $75.00. Some have a set price for a service, like locating the most suitable care facility or making a home safety assessment.

After reviewing Mom's current health status, medications, and appointments, all of which we had kept filed in a notebook in the kitchen, and a discussion of Mom's daily routine, Louise made a couple of suggestions. The first one was easy enough to handle: my mom and I both agreed it would be a good idea if Louise would drop by for regular monthly visits, to check in on how things were going. She wanted to hear how Mom was doing with her physical therapy that had been recommended to help improve her balance and could check her medication changes, take her blood pressure, and check on her healing wounds. (Mom had fallen and cut her knees a month or so before I came and had needed lots of stitches.) Louise would also talk with Mom about her medications. She encouraged Mom to use her cane around the house and suggested a rolling cart or walker as an even better alternative. I would speak to Louise after her visits by phone and get filled in on Mom's progress. Better still, Louise would be on call in case I wanted her to check in on Mom in between her regular visits. Mom agreed that having the same nurse who knew her history would be a good idea, especially in an emergency.

The second suggestion was a little harder to accept: Louise recommended to both of us that while Mom was recovering and getting her medications adjusted, she could use some extra help around the house. She urged us to consider hiring a home health aide from a local home health agency; she even had the name of a worker there whom she thought would get on well with Mom. Home health workers need to be affiliated with a certified home health agency in order to qualify for reimbursement from a few private insurers who cover it. I hadn't known that and, in fact, I had forgotten about that long-term care policy Mom had been paying for all those years. Turns out, her long-term care policy would pay for her home-health aides under certain circumstances. Right there, I felt Louise had more than paid back the cost of her consultation.

When big changes are about to take place, it always helps to hear firsthand stories from those who have undergone similar experiences. Louise had used this local home health agency when her husband became ill and needed a home aide. She shared how her husband had not wanted a stranger in the house, but had soon become quite chummy with his caregiver and relied on her for so many things that Louise had previously had done for him. Having a firsthand account from someone who had used these services went a long way to reassuring me that hiring a home health aide might be just the thing to get Mom back on her feet (and me back home.) My mother, on the other hand, was not so keen on the idea.

While Louise sat and chatted with Mom, I admired her skill at connecting with my mother's hopes and fears. With her straightforward "matter of fact" manner, she was chatting comfortably about subjects my mother had dismissed as ridiculous whenever I tried to raise them, such as driving, using her cane or walker or her diet. Louise's care and deep experience seemed to allow my mom to come to terms with a life that, while it might not be exactly what she had in mind, was certainly better than many of the alternatives.

Accepting the Help

While Mom had seemed to see the valid points Louise was making about letting go of some of her accustomed pleasures, like driving herself and preparing all her meals, she remained unconvinced on the issue of having a stranger in her home to help out on a regular basis. Mom really liked her time alone and was adamant about not having anyone in the house all day, every day. "It's only half a day," I reminded her, "and only three days a week. You will have your time alone, even more because I won't be here all the time and knowing that you have help I can go back to my house."

But that was not the point to my mother. She had a picture in her head about how life was supposed to be and she was determined to stick to her role in the movie. This meant she lived alone and asked no one for help. She drove to the post office every day, the grocery and library every week, and to her hairdresser every other week and she didn't want anybody else in the picture. Clearly, the fact that I had been sitting in the front row for these six weeks past didn't count, clearly I wasn't officially in her movie.

Over and over again, I would lay out the case for getting help. I was confident reason would prevail because I was clearly right about this. Mom would counter with her side of the story. Her "facts" seemed skewed to me, but that's what she thought about mine, so we arrived at an impasse every time. Just when I thought we were making progress, she would rally and point out just how capable she was, and, to be fair, she did have some good points. Mom had managed very well without help up to now (never mind the falls) so why not carry on?

I was at my wits' end. I thought back to some of the insights Louise had shared with me. "Often older parents do not want their kids dictating rules to them," Louise explained. "But because a care manager is a professional and has a different approach, aged parents often accept our advice, for example, like making changes in lifestyles, such as getting home helpers, or making the home safer, or getting physical therapy, or giving up driving." The point is that having an outside expert make the case for these tough changes takes the burden off of the family. "I tell my clients that it is a gift to your children to let them know what you want, in terms of care, and to accept help when needed," says Louise.

I decided to keep pointing out the advantages of some help around the house, and to go looking for ways to fund this help, should Mom agree to take on a helper. I figured it would pay off eventually if Mom fell again or had some other crisis, and had to admit she couldn't manage on her own anymore.

What actually constitutes a crisis? Good question. One way health care workers answer that is to assess the ability of an elderly patient to perform daily tasks that most of us can do on our own. But which tasks? The insurance companies and the government seem to have agreed on a list of the six critical activities of daily life (ADL) that are necessary for basic independent living. The rule is that the loss of any two of the ADLs will trigger the need for some kind of assistance, which in turn triggers the payouts to you from your long-term care insurance so you have money to pay for care. Once a doctor or a health care worker has certified that a senior has lost two ADLs, your aged relative can apply for payments from long-term care policies. Some seniors can even qualify for extra cash from several government programs.

Six Critical Activities of Daily Living

1. **Bathing** - sponge bath, tub or shower; no assistance except with one part of the body
2. **Dressing** - gets clothes and dresses without assistance except for tying shoes
3. **Toilet** - goes to toilet room, uses toilet, arranges clothes and returns without assistance
4. **Transferring** - gets in and out of bed without help
5. **Continence** - controls bowel and bladder completely by self without occasional accidents
6. **Feeding** - feeds self without assistance except for help cutting meat and buttering bread

Getting an Eldercare Attorney

Thanks to Louise, I realized that Mom should investigate other sources of income to help defray her necessary health care costs, and she put us in touch with an attorney who specializes in eldercare. I wanted to be sure I was not burning any bridges or leaving any options unexplored in my quest to fund care for my mother. I was looking for funding from Mom's long-term care policy, and possibly the veterans administration, since my father had been a veteran of WWII, and I heard they give out pensions to spouses in need. If all else failed, I knew there was always Medicaid in the far distant and very broke future. I was hoping it wouldn't come to that, as I knew by now how much that would limit the choices for care.

I found a very helpful book called <u>How to Protect Your Family's Assets from Devastating Nursing Home Costs</u> by K. Gabriel Heiser, an attorney, that answered many of my questions and left me more determined than ever to get a plan in place for all eventualities for my mother. I would worry about myself later, when all this was settled.

Louise, our care manager, gave me the name of two lawyers in my mom's area who specialized in geriatric law and she gave me a personal recommendation for one of the two. It was good to know someone who had firsthand knowledge about the professional I would be consulting. Please note that the law is different state to state, so you need to consult an attorney in the state where your loved one resides for accurate information.

In our first conversation with the eldercare attorney, which we arranged as a phone meeting, I quickly explained our situation and what kind of questions I had for him. I also asked him to please alert me to any pitfalls I had not foreseen. (Notes I had already forwarded to him included my mom's lists of assets and the possible cost of several levels of care.)

The attorney raised a number of points that were pertinent to our particular situation that I had not considered, and thus it was a very worthwhile investment. He helped me understand the qualification for being awarded a pension for spouses of combat veterans from the Veterans Administration. The rules require that the surviving spouse meet the government's main criteria for health care assistance, meaning that she needs to be short two ADLs. There is no minimum income level to qualify. If you are a widow/widower of a veteran, and you have health care issues, you should look into it. You or your spouse earned this pension for providing service for your country and the VA wants you to have it if you qualify. The people in the application office were extremely helpful and you can find out more about this benefit on the Veterans Administration website: www.va.gov.

The lawyer then explained how to handle the family home, what property would disqualify us for Medicaid if it came to that. Most of all, this information helped us to make a clear, honest, and concise picture of Mom's medical and financial qualifications for the present as well as the future claims when applying for long-term care benefits, pensions, and possibly Medicaid in the future, if the need arose. It is vital to research any financial moves for their future impact. You can qualify for one benefit that disqualifies you from another. For instance, giving away assets by putting the family home in someone else's name is a poor strategy as there is a "look back" period for Medicaid to prevent fraud. One can, however, spend money on making the home safer and more suitable for the elderly person to "age in place." In many cases, this expense can be counted as a medically necessary loss and thus may be deducted from one's income for tax purposes.

With his help, we figured that it was more beneficial for us to borrow against the value of Mom's home to pay for needed renovations than to apply for a reverse mortgage. It was better for us because it saved money in the long run, however, it is dependent on the value of your home, equity in your home and the amount needed. You really need to get all your information together and then get the advice of a professional to determine your most beneficial and legal way to proceed.

Old and Paying for It

While Mom and I danced around this issue of home health care, I called Mom's doctors for their opinions. They advised me that it was probably not wise to leave Mom on her own right now. She could feed herself, finding her mouth with a fork, but because of her diminished eyesight, it was a challenge for her to prepare nutritious food for herself since her macular degeneration, made her vision very bad indeed. She was legally blind in one eye and had "low vision" in the other, even with glasses. Mom had hidden this dramatic loss of vision very well. She used a magnifying glass for many things now, but I had assumed she was reading things that had really, really small print! It is hard to cook with a big magnifying glass in one hand and your cane in the other.

Then there was bathing, her legs were too rickety to allow her to get in and out of the bathtub safely, and more falls seemed inevitable. Mom had been giving herself sponge baths for the last few weeks because of the bandaged cuts on her knees from a previous fall, but that was not a long-term solution to the hygiene issue. The doctors were concerned that if I had to go home and there was no other friend or relative available to help out around the house, Mom would not recover her strength and might even start to lose weight again. The doctors agreed that having a home health aide was a good solution to keeping Mom safe, recovering, and comfortable in her own home.

Finding the Money

To get the ball rolling, I read over Mom's long-term care policy. She kept it in the metal lock box with all her paperwork, next to the receipts for monthly expenses neatly stacked and banded in the kitchen cupboard. Mom was great at this. No one would ever accuse her of slipping in the mind if they saw how she could lay her hand on any paper needed, however far in the past it had been generated.

It made me think about my own desk back home and wonder that if I ever fell ill, how my kids would manage. I started to worry that they would never find the contact information for my insurance policies, or even my will for that matter. I vowed then and there to get my affairs in order as soon as I got home, though when that would happen I could not tell.

The first step to getting her long-term insurer to begin to pay out on Mom's policy was to prove she had a physical need for home health aide help. Mom's concierge doc did the honors and filled in the form for the long-term care benefits. It was hand-scrawled, and none too legible, but he ticked off the two ADL boxes, eating and bathing, and I

Eldercare Attorney

Here are a few questions to ask when trying to find a good eldercare attorney:

- How long has he or she been practicing?
- Is elder law the person's specialty?
- How much of the person's practice is involved with elder law?
- Is there an initial consultation fee?

Most lawyers will have no problem answering these kinds of questions. If someone tries to brush these off, it may be a sign of a poor fit. If you are uncomfortable with the answers you get, keep looking. You want to start off with someone who you feel has the experience and knowledge to keep your loved one's best interests in mind.

Elder law encompasses many different fields of law. The National Academy of Elder Law Attorneys website (www.naela.org) lists some of these:

- Preservation/transfer of assets seeking to avoid spousal impoverishment when a spouse enters a nursing home
- Medicaid
- Medicare claims and appeals
- Social Security and disability claims and appeals
- Supplemental and long-term health insurance issues
- Disability planning, including use of durable powers of attorney, living trusts, "living wills," for financial management and health-care decisions, and other means of delegating management and decision-making to another in case of incompetency or incapacity
- Conservatorships and guardianships
- Estate planning, including planning for the management of one's estate during life and its disposition on death through the use of trusts, wills, and other planning documents
- Probate
- Administration and management of trusts and estates

- Long-term care placements in nursing home and life care communities
- Nursing home issues including questions of patients' rights and nursing home quality
- Elder abuse and fraud recovery cases
- Housing issues, including discrimination and home equity conversions
- Age discrimination in employment
- Retirement, including public and private retirement benefits, survivor benefits, and pension benefits
- Health law
- Mental health law

Figure out what your special concerns are, and then ask your prospective attorney if these areas are their usual area of practice. Lawyer's fees vary widely. Some may charge by the hour, while others may charge a specific fee for a set of services. Discuss fees before hiring an elder law attorney and make sure you get an agreement in writing. Keep your other family members informed that you are seeking a consultation. Invite them to come along and share the advice you have been given. Before you meet with your lawyer, put together your lists of important data. The Family Caregiver Alliance (www.caregiver.org) and other caregiver organizations have put together lists of information and documents you may need to bring to your attorney's attention, such as the following:

- List of major assets, including real property, stocks, cash, and valuable objects such as jewelry
- List of all major debts
- Copies of deeds, stock certificates, mortgages and the like that show ownership names of the assets and how the titles are held
- Any major contracts the person may have signed
- Copies of wills and/or powers of attorney
- List of bank-held assets, such as cash, CDs, and safe deposit boxes

Long-Term Care Insurance

Mary bought her own long-term care insurance (LTC) when she saw how important her mother's policy was to her comfort and care in these past few years. People who have not had to take care of a loved one don't know how important LTC insurance can be. They think they will just spend all their money so then the government will take care of them. It is not as easy as that.

Mary spoke with Ginny Kintz, an independent insurance agent who specializes in Long-Term Care Insurance with years of experience in this relatively new field. She shared her knowledge and experience, saying:

"I found that almost eighty-five percent of the people I talk to have called me because they have had someone who needed LTC. They watched this person who is dear to them go through all their money and ended up having to live in a place they do not like, a place they did not choose."

There is such a variety of continuing-care facilities that it is hard to find just the right combination of care and community. Some Continuing Care Retirement Communities (CCRC) are quite wonderful. They look like a college campus. They have apartments or cottages for independent living, and there is assisted living or nursing care. You know where you will be and how you will be cared for should your health change. There are different variations of payment structures with CCRC's, with different prices depending on your budget. One thing they have in common is a requirement to be in relatively good health upon entering. In spite of a wide range of fees for these places, they cost more than you ever imagined they would. Having a Long-Term Care Policy can make all the difference because once you need it, it will give you monthly checks that you can use to pay for your care.

Ginny said, "A good LTC policy, if designed properly, can cover all the LTC costs of the different levels of care, so you never have to worry about paying."

Mary says "when I bought my policy, I was concerned about the amount of cash I would need to keep me in style, so I made sure I got enough coverage for a fine decline!" You can check out Ginny's website (www.kintzltc.com) for a free downloadable booklet that explains all the LTC options. There is also a federal website that has a tool to help you figure out the cost of care in your own area: www.ltcfeds.com. That can be your guide to how much LTC insurance you need in your geographic area. You can also check out www.medicare.gov for cost comparisons on the different kind of communities by state.

Ginny stated that the average length of stay in a nursing home for a woman is 3.0 years, and for a man it is 2.5 years. For assisted living, or a nursing home, the average stay is eighteen months. It is so short because people usually only go to a nursing home when they need skilled care. For example, the average yearly cost for nursing care in Virginia is $87,000.00. In New Hampshire, the cost is $93,000.00. At that rate, most people would burn through their estates pretty fast! Even if skilled nursing care may not be necessary, it is likely an older person will need some form of assistance to keep him or her healthy and safe, such as home health aides or housekeeping services.

There will be so many more people needing care as our population ages. Twelve thousand people a day turn sixty-five, and that will be the case for the next twenty years! Ginny states: "To me, that is not the most amazing fact about long-term care. The most amazing fact is that thirty-nine percent of the people needing long-term care are younger than sixty-five! Accidents, Parkinson's disease, and stroke impact people of all ages. People need to remember that they could need this care, at any age, not just because they are getting old."

So you might need to use your policy before age sixty five, for example, if you had a skiing accident. After you get out of the hospital from an injury, you could face six months of rehab and that could be covered by your LTC policy. If you are a woman and you make it to the age if sixty-five, your odds of needing long-term care, that's care for longer than ninety days, are one in two. If you are a man, the odds are one in three.

Those are phenomenal odds. It is much more likely that you will use your LTC policy than you will your homeowners or car insurance! Everyone who can should buy Long-Term Care insurance, but not everyone can qualify now. You have to be relatively healthy to even get LTC insurance. You should get your policy as early as age forty because the rate will be lower, and once you have it, you cannot be dropped as long as you pay your premiums.

The three things people want to know about LTC are:
- What does it cover?

   A set number of days at full care is translated into a dollar amount
- How much does it cost?

   Premiums are based on your age and health at time of purchase
- When should I buy it?

   The younger and more healthy you are, the less you will pay for your policy!

Ginny: "The hardest thing to get across to people is that they probably will need care. Denial is the hardest hurdle I have to overcome in providing LTC planning, and it is especially prevalent in baby boomers! Most of us think it can't happen here. We believe we will live hale and hearty until we keel over dead. Most people think 'old age' is fifteen years older than they are right now! Yet people plan for car accidents and natural disasters much better than they are planning for needing some help as they age. Just knowing you are far more likely to need care as you age, than for any of these other more common insurance purchases, is a good first step."

Many people want to protect their assets for future generations and most people want to avoid being dependent on others. Long-Term

Care Insurance is a way to achieve both. "Some people think they have enough money, they can afford not to buy LTC insurance, but they really do not understand that 'enough' could mean they have five million dollars of readily available cash on hand. Most people don't, but many high net worth people who do have that kind of cash have LTC insurance because it just makes good sense to transfer the risk to an insurance company. There is nothing so delightful as having someone else write you a check for $10,000 a month rather than writing it yourself!"

Mary's mother bought her policy a decade ago and spent a big percentage of her income to pay for it. She was happy to make the sacrifice to ensure her care, and Mary was so grateful she did ten years later when that policy made a big difference to her. Things have changed in the industry since then, that is why it is important for people to buy their policies now, while they still qualify.

I asked Ginny how to decide the best level of LTC insurance to buy.

"First, they should look at the cost of nursing care in their region. The average stay is about three years, so multiply the rate times at least three years. Then decide the deductible you want, usually between twenty and one hundred and eighty days. This is stated in days, not dollars. Keep in mind that Medicare may pay up to the first one hundred days of skilled nursing care. This is because LTC was originally set up to dovetail with Medicare, which will cover twenty to one hundred days depending on the reason for hospitalization. Consider that along with your ability to cover the deductible. Once you have satisfied this deductible one time, it goes away for the rest of your life." Choose a big deductible to lower the monthly cost but only if you can easily afford it.

"The next thing to decide is how large a "pot of money" you want in your policy. Don't buy too much. You will want to buy more than you think you will need. So if the average life expectancy with full care is four years, you want to get five years coverage. Multiply the daily maximum payout by the length of coverage and you have the dollar value

Looking back, the picture is so much clearer. Now I can see where I failed to pick up on some important clues. First, when my brother called and asked that I come down to see Mom's condition for myself, he gave me a very dire picture of her condition, and although I thought my brother to be an exaggerator of exceptional skill, I was impressed by his distress. And so I went down immediately. What I didn't quite understand was his deep desire that his assessment be wrong, and if he was right, his deep desire, indeed his belief, that I could make it all go away.

As I had left my magic wand at home, I could do neither. I have to admire my brother for succeeding at communication where I failed. In that one phone call, he had conveyed such a sense of urgency that I felt the need for action. My phone style was the exact opposite. My phone calls to him were calm reports about Mom's conditions and intellectual discussions of diagnoses and remedies. Instead of pulling the fire alarm, it was as if I was going room to room whispering that, if you didn't mind, could you please evacuate the building because it was, ah, on fire—not a lot, just a tad. No wonder he never got my sense of urgency!

He was focused on these strangers suddenly tromping through our mother's house. Who were these people? What if they made things worse? What if they took advantage of Mom? What if they just came over and watched TV and pilfered her treasures? Perhaps because my brother had not seen the need for daily if not hourly help and had not found the solution himself, he was not willing to accept my solution as a good one.

How to Hire an Aide

You can hire a trusted friend or someone that has been recommended to you, or go through an agency for a home health aide. There are a few reasons why you might want to hire your caregiver through a state-certified agency. Because we went through an agency to find our home health aide, she had been given a thorough background check and was bonded. Aides from an agency are forbidden to accept gifts of any kind from the care recipients, unless they pass through the agency for approval. In addition, they are not to perform any care that might be construed as medical. Even trimming nails is forbidden. They receive training for helping the care recipient to bathe with dignity, as well as guidelines for proper nutrition and food safety. Should there be any dissatisfaction with the aide, one has only to call the agency to get a replacement. There is no question of hiring and firing an individual. Tax issues are handled by the agency. Should your caregiver need a day off, the agency will supply a replacement if rescheduling is not possible.

The agency also provided help with filling out the needed forms for the VA and LTC insurance company, ensuring an approval on the first try. Eventually, I was able to have them bill the insurance company directly for payment for our home help, thus eliminating a lot of paperwork.

Hiring private aides can work out well as long as you have good references. Tracey liked the local help she found for her mother—people they had known for years. They treated her mom with tender care and, as the family were paying for the care themselves, it was a fine way to go.

I was relieved to be on my way home, secure in the knowledge that my mom was in good hands, as safe as I could make her for now. The minute my car crossed the line into my

Networks of Friends and Support

According to the Administration on Aging, a federal agency, In 2000, approximately 605 million people were 60 years or older. By 2050, that number is expected to be close to 2 billion. It should come as no surprise that by the year 2020, the US will need more caregivers than teachers. Many caregivers will be the friends and family of those needing care and they may not even consider themselves to be caregivers. One estimate has it that seventy-five percent of caregivers are unpaid. The average age of a caregiver is sixty-three.

Fifty-nine to seventy-nine percent of the caregivers are women, many not so young themselves when they are called to step in and care for a husband or parent. It seems to be expected of them. The stress from providing this care is mental, emotional, and physical. Having a network of support is vital to keep you sane and geared up for this venture. For many caregivers, it is a big surprise to find that their often heroic efforts will go unrecognized, and may even be criticized by those receiving care. **Here are five tips** for putting together a support network:

1. Find an ear

Every caregiver needs a support network. If you do not have a friend or clergy member to whom you can bare your soul, I recommend seeing a psychological counselor of some kind. If you just can't see your way clear to do that, go online and google caregivers network, caregivers support, etc., and your location. You will find the usual collection of people and businesses ready to take your money, but be persistent and you will find a local group that may be able to give you more than moral support.

Feel like this is too much to tackle? I'm not surprised. Many caregivers feel so drained by day's end that they can do little more for themselves than fall into bed, where they will probably not sleep that well, for keeping an ear out for their charge. In that case, go online to this website: http://www.caregiversupportnetwork.org. Read some of the massages sent by caregivers. I guarantee you will feel like you have found out where the rest of the people on this "planet caregiving" are hiding. You can vent here and get some judgment-free commiseration from your fellow caregivers. There is a place to look up specifics—type in the word "stress!" It is a rich vein. This simple act of hearing the same experiences from others will drain off some of your isolation. You may even strike up a friendship with people you "meet" there who are in your same situation. Whatever you do, keep trying until you have a good ear and shoulder to cry on.

2. Acknowledge yourself for your contribution

Step two is to recognize your own contribution. It is massive! The love, energy, and devotion it takes to care for a loved one is enormous. Give yourself a pat on the back. You are on the front lines here. Never mind you cannot keep your composure; you are doing good work.

3. Find ways to support your own health and well-being

You absolutely MUST take care of yourself if you are to care for someone else. Remember what they say on airplanes when you get the safety lecture? Put on your own oxygen mask before helping others. It will do your loved one absolutely no good if you fall down from stress and can't help them anymore. Caring for yourself is your first step to caring for your loved one.

- Get respite help (your geriatric care manager can direct you to resources) so you can have a few hours to yourself.
- Pay attention to your own nutrition, don't stress eat, make a good diet plan and stick to it.
- Get some exercise; even if all you can do is to take a few minutes to stretch. Try to set aside thirty minutes a day to do yoga, or find a good aerobics TV show.
- Get silly! I find humor helps when I am stressed. Read a funny book or watch a funny movie.

them take him to his house "to check on it" and he went in and up and down the stairs. When I went to get him the next day to take him home for good, he was still angry. Now mad and saying, "I went home, I went up and down the stairs with no problem, why did I come here? They've done nothing for me!"

And that is when I lost it, "Why didn't you just stay at your house?" I asked in a rage. He looked at me blankly as if I was crazy. "I'm sorry you have to suffer so much, that you have been forced to live in this place!" waving my arm around indicating the luxury apartment that he was in (the best the area has to offer!). "I'm sorry that it bothers you so much to have me care and worry about you!" He maintained his belligerence and anger, so he checked out of rehab that day and I drove him home, made his lunch and left him there with his ninety-three-year-old friend who had come to visit!

The following day when I called to check in with him he sounded quiet and tired when he answered the phone. "How's it going, Dad?" I asked. "Terrible. I haven't had a meal in two days" he responded sadly. "Dad, didn't you have breakfast? I left you quiche for breakfast. I made you lunch and dinner yesterday, didn't you eat it?" He seemed confused and I was shocked at his change in demeanor and rushed over to his house to find him dozing in his recliner, the ice packs on his knee. I realized that he was still getting the anesthesia out of his system; the narcotics he was taking for pain were affecting his short term memory. He knew he had been in the hospital and remembered some things but had no recall of much of the time he was there.

I made him some meals, sorted out his refrigerator, and went shopping for him. We called the VNA and arranged home visits with the nurses. Things began to fall in to place, but even after two weeks he didn't realize that my sister and I had been to see him every day in the hospital and at home.

The worst came about two weeks after his surgery when he told me that he had "no expectations" of me. "What do you mean, no expectations? You don't want me to care about what happens to you?" I asked confused. "I have no expectations." he said flatly. He wouldn't elaborate and I was left to figure out what he meant. So many possibilities. Is it that he doesn't want me to worry about him, or that he doesn't want me to physically take care of him, or that he doesn't want me to take away his independence?

And then the real meaning of his words came out. "What do you think I am, a decrepit old man who can't take care of himself anymore?" he asked scrunching his face and shaking his fists. "Well, no, Dad, but you are acting like that! You need help right now. I don't want you to fall down the stairs and lie here alone for three days." And so he finally took the advice of the visiting nurses and got himself an Alert bracelet only to return it to the company once his knee was fully recovered. "What if you fall now?" I asked. "Oh, I'll be all right," he said.

What my dad went through after his knee surgery is what doctors now call a postoperative "acute confusional state." After surgery, elderly patients often get disoriented from the pain medicine and can experience delirium, or suddenly become very aggressive or have acute panic attacks. The ability of the kidneys of an eighty-five-year-old patient to clear out anesthesia is going to be very different than a forty-year-old. "To me the most important treatment of post surgical delirium is having a family member with you," says Dr. Leo Cooney, Chief of Geriatrics at Yale New Haven Hospital. "I think that gets you through it a lot better than Haldol or restraints or anything else. I think that you being with your parent in the hospital is the best treatment for when they get confused. And they are going to get confused, particularly with morphine. I mean, it is always a balancing act, you don't want them in pain, pain is not good for you but there are cognitive effects of analgesic medication."

Dad recovered fully from his knee replacement, often showing people how nicely his scar looks and how well he can bend his knee without pain now! Either he does not remember those weeks in recovery or has chosen to forget, it doesn't really matter anymore, he is my dad and I have him back for a while.

Driving

How to decide when it's time to give up the keys!

Tracey's dad is still driving. His ten-year-old Prius has bumps and bruises on all four corners. That is a sign it is time to stop driving. Once he backed out of his garage with the door open and bent it almost off. Once he fell asleep driving home from the VA hospital which is a one-and–one-half-hour drive, which he insists that he can still do by himself. We let him do it; we are too busy to drive him. Dad was a pilot, and was flying until age seventy-nine when he voluntarily stopped flying. Smart guy. When will he know it is time to stop driving? When will we have to tell him he has to?

Now that he has had his cataracts removed, his vision is back to 20-20. He went and got a new driving license that says he doesn't need glasses to drive. They only had him do the eye test for his new license. When will they do a road test with him again? Who and how are these decisions made? Every state has different laws about when people have to stop driving and how frequently actual behind-the-wheel testing is done.

Tracey says, "When my daughters told me their grandma was using her hand to lift her leg so her foot could go from the gas pedal to brake, I knew it was time to talk with Mom about driving." Mom even admitted there were a couple times she couldn't move her foot off the gas pedal to the brake quick enough and that was the end of that. She willingly gave up driving, gave her car to my daughter, and the hunt for regular drivers began."

Have you ever caught yourself talking out loud to the elderly driver in front of you as they hesitate and slowly turn around lamp posts in the parking lot, looking for the perfect space? Patience can run thin, but consider what a good thing it is that many elderly drivers use more caution. They know their reaction times are slower, their vision less acute, even if they won't admit it to you. Losing the keys to the car means more than entering a more relaxed time of life, being driven all over town in a chauffeured car. It means the loss of freedom the elderly depend on for their way of life. Often the cascade of events around the loss of this mobility in our society - a society that is built around an automobile - is devastating.

Still, it is a fact that *more* older drivers than younger ones are likely to be in multiple car accidents, especially at intersections. At age sixty-five, the risk begins to increase, and at age seventy, the risk of driver fatality rises sharply. The fatality rate for drivers eighty-five and over is nine times as high as the rate for drivers twenty-five through sixty-nine years old, according to AAA.

Even though you may want to support your elderly friend or relative to drive as long as possible, you probably worry about their driving abilities. We don't all retain the ability to drive a car throughout our lifetime. Physical disabilities, mental illness, medications, loss of vision, or frailty can end anyone's driving career at any age.

Great tact is required when broaching this topic. Before you do, think through the daily routine of the older person you care about and try to come up with alternative solutions to the dilemma of being stranded without their car. They may feel trapped by their loss of control over their schedule and afraid they will lose the joy of spontaneity in their life.

Getting a third-party evaluation may be a good idea. Start with the family doctor, but keep in mind that they may be reluctant to recommend a surrender of the keys. Mary's mother's doctors would not come out with a definitive "no way" on the driving issue, even though she was legally blind in one eye and had what is known as "low vision" in the other, even with glasses. Doctors may feel they have to pick their battles and, as this is not a medical issue, they will want someone else to take the lead in the matter of giving up the keys. Getting the physical facts from them is a good start, however.

Only when you are sure about the good alternatives for your elder driver, have the medical facts in hand, and are feeling calm and centered should you bring up the topic of driving. Looking over the AAA site section on senior driving might be a good start (www.aaa.com). AAA has three assessment tools for older drivers and some good support to improve the driving skills of those deemed safe on the road. One is a self evaluation, another is an interactive one, and the third is a professional assessment.

Your senior driver may have had their own doubts about their abilities, so beginning with the alternative transportation methods might be a good start. No one wants to come out and say they are failing at something they have done all their life, but with enough support and time, they may be able to adopt the idea of not driving and make it seem like it was their own idea.

Living Will

This is one task on your list to secure a happy, old age for yourself and your loved ones you hope you won't need, but will be very glad you made the effort if you do. Sure, it may seem depressing to contemplate all the awful possibilities, but how much worse would it be if you did not have the living will in place? Much worse. It matters, so just do it! This is one of the cheap things you can accomplish that will give you peace of mind.

A living will is a legal document that provides instructions for others to make medical care decisions for you when you are no longer able to make medical decisions for yourself. A healthcare agent, sometimes called a healthcare proxy, patient advocate, surrogate, or healthcare representative may also be appointed in advance to make medical care decisions when you are not able to make decisions and healthcare choices for yourself.

A living will states what type of care you will allow, and not allow, should you become unable to make medical decisions. A copy of this document should be given to your primary doctor and to the person you designate as your medical proxy. That person is usually a relative or very close friend who you grant permission to make medical decisions on your behalf should you be unable to. This person is your designated point person for your care. Their job is to honor the wishes you stated in your living will. Mary and Tracey believe this person should not be one or all of your children. Spare them this task and trust someone who has a clear idea of your wishes and who shares your values about life and death.

Why do you need a living will?

- To avoid legal wrangling
- To prevent suffering
- To spare your finances
- To give you the peace of mind that comes with control

How do you do it?

- You can get the forms online for free or cheap and fill them in yourself, or go to your own attorney. Get them notarized and file a copy where you keep all your precious documents.
- Leave a list of these documents where they are easily seen (on your desk) and tell your near and dear ones where it is.
- Tell your doctor you have a living will and give him a copy.
- There are different forms for each state; get one from your primary residence state.
- Medical options to prevent death are becoming more numerous by the day.

Your doctors want to preserve life; it is their job. Consider adding a customized paragraph to your living will (that you and your health-care proxy both sign) giving this person broad interpretation powers to block emergency measures that are not specifically listed in your living will. The health-care proxy has the power to prevent any action that would prolong your life. You need someone who can definitively order the medical professionals to honor your wishes. Take the case of *New York Magazine* (May 28, 2012) author Michael Wolff's mother who has serious dementia and was given, unbeknownst to family members, massive doses of anti-seizure medication after what had appeared to be a stroke, in spite of her do not resuscitate (DNR) orders. Your proxy needs to ask about all medications and gets to say *yes* or *no*.

What do you have to decide?

Think about being permanently unconscious or in intractable pain, but having health care professionals come in and do these things to you—things that will prolong your life just when you are going about the business of letting go of life.

home. All the familiar old furnishings probably looked fine to Mom, but coming in with fresh eyes, everything looked dowdy, cumbersome, a potential threat to her health and well-being. There were loose throw rugs, dusty sofas and chairs long past needing a re-upholstery job, sharp-edged marble coffee tables, and rickety chairs. Suddenly, everywhere I looked I saw potential concussions, cuts, trips, and falls. We tend to have dramatic imaginations in my family and with time on my hands, I might have gotten carried away by my own dark vision.

Realizing I needed just a bit of tact, I started off small, bringing out the paint samples and making forays out to stores for fabrics and carpet squares. Together we chose a new palette for the living room which Mom admitted could use a fresh coat of paint. I pointed out that the drapes had been in place for thirty years and had surely paid for themselves by now. Time for some fresh choices!

Mom seemed anxious about making some of these decisions and there was a note of, "Yes, we could do that, but . . ." that let me know she was not wanting these changes, however much she seemed to agree with me. As we chatted about which chairs were really needed and where they might be shifted to instead, I realized that all the strategic placement of the furniture that looked so wrong to my young eyes had a secondary purpose for Mom. They were not there to sit on but to be used as handholds. For the first time I watched, really watched, as Mom moved slowly and carefully from chair to kitchen and saw that the decor had evolved from one of beauty to practicality, accommodating Mom's need for support as she moved through her home. The thick white carpet might be luxurious underfoot, but to Mom, who had trouble lifting her feet at every step, it posed a hazard (I saw) that had to be carefully accounted for by moving from handhold to handhold to get across the room.

This was going to be more of a challenge than I thought, realizing that the shiny hunter green rolling cart I had ordered from Costco and my niece had decorated with Mom's name and a handy cup holder had gone unused for a reason. There was no space to push it through these rooms full of furniture and, to Mom, no need for it, as her method of subtly slipping from one grip on a chair back to table, to door jam, and so into the kitchen and the island for support was working just fine. Now I understood why she resisted even the smallest change! Her furniture was exactly where she needed it to be. If I took away the tall chair that looked to be clogging the passage from bedroom to laundry nook, she would have nothing to grip, no support at all. Now I understood all the falls and weird furniture placements.

No wonder she resisted outings! Her cane, while useful, was really not enough support for her balance-challenged posture these days. At home, Mom could maintain her dignity and stay upright, but not always as the recent falls had shown. I thought back to how the clutter had appeared, one piece at a time, and realized she had asked the cleaning lady to move a bookcase or desk into each spot where she had lost her footing until she had what looked to her like a safe path to where she needed to go. I now saw why she worked so hard to conceal the number and frequency of these tumbles, calling first one relative, then another and swearing all to secrecy so as to "not worry the children."

The problem, I realized in retrospect, was not concern for her safety; she too, was concerned. The difference came in exactly how that concern would be addressed. In her mind, Mom had done a masterful job of "making do" and creating a safe, secure home for herself. To me, it looked like a cluttered death trap, no wonder she resisted the smallest change. Shifting the placement of one chair might result in a serious fall!

The other problem was that to Mom, the use of a cane, and then a "walker," as she called her rolling cart, represented a loss of dignity. They were signs that she was "failing" and that was mortifying to her. "Do you think I am just a batty little old woman?" she would ask when

I insisted she take her cane into the grocery store. "I have my own ways, why can't you leave me be?" She refused to believe that she needed any of these kinds of "safety" aids. She was fine, thank you very much. And no, she did not need to use a walker!

At the grocery store I had to admit, she had a point. Mom directed me to park out by the cart corral, instead of in the handicapped spot for which she was qualified. Then she nimbly got out of the car, eased her way around the back, using the car for support until she got her hands on a shopping cart, then slowly, but quite steadily, she made her stately way into and around the store. I am not quite sure how she managed getting the bags into the house without me, but I could see why she had stopped buying spring water by the gallon! I left that conversation for another day.

With my new realizations, I was more determined than ever to clear the decks and make Mom's home a showplace of safety and beauty. I found myself turning into a master negotiator, or so I thought. I persuaded Mom that a flatter carpet with a tight weave would be much easier to navigate. "The carpet in here needs replacing, but in the dining room and parlor, it is like new! I don't want to rip that up; it would be a waste!" Mom replied, setting me back a bit, for she was right! I plunged ahead anyway, "We could have the floors re-done after the whole house is painted inside; won't it be nice to have everything all fresh?" See how I did that? I went from speaking about sprucing up the living room to vacating the house and redecorating from top to bottom. Before long I was talking about replacing the old brown cabinets in the bathrooms, putting down real tile instead of the linoleum, and making a walk-in shower out of her spare closet.

Mom sat in her recliner (the fat, overstuffed, fading, beige recliner that was going to get pitched in favor of a sleek, new, reclining wing chair, if I had any say in the matter) and said she just didn't know; maybe the improvements were needed, but maybe she could make do— and how would she pay for all this?

My brother came down for the weekend and I shared my sketches and swatches with him. He actually had built the house thirty years before when he was starting out as a contractor and he agreed an update was just what we needed. The fixtures and finishes he had put in to start with were really not top quality, just what Mom and Dad could afford at the time. He had always thought to upgrade. Before I knew it, he was talking about replacing all the windows and breaking through the dining room wall. New decks, kitchen counters, and a big gas barbecue went on the list, and Mom was left out of this conversation entirely, for we both knew what she would say to our grand plans.

All this fine rebuilding of Mom's world would take time and money, neither of which was in ready supply for any of us at the time, so we put away the sketches for another day and settled on a bathroom remodel followed by a paint and carpet replacement. These seemed the best choices to improve Mom's safety and enjoyment. We both mourned the lost opportunity for the new windows that would open up the view to Bridge Creek, the granite kitchen counters and new cabinets. On the bright side, we had found just enough money for these needed improvements and we were prepared to start off slowly.

Mom reluctantly agreed. We never told her that the money for this first round of home rehab was coming from the accounts she had started in each of our names after she and Dad retired. How astonishing to learn that while making budget-oriented choices in their new home, Mom had set up these accounts for us, so that some of her small retirement income would go automatically to a fund for the two of us.

Mom and I picked out the new bathroom tile, grout, paint, and cabinets for the guest bathroom. We decided to give the local contractor chosen by my brother a try with this small job and see how he did. Mom would stay for a week at my brother's house while the work went on and then return home for the unveiling.

and polish. Add a plant or some cut flowers and you will be amazed at how good you feel spending time there now.

3. Clear clutter from your bedroom

Bedrooms often gather clutter first because we stow stuff there, often to make the public areas of the house more presentable. You spend more time sleeping than doing any other activity in your home. The quality of your sleep is directly affected by the condition of your bedroom. It's hard to sleep well when your bedroom clutter is crying out for order.

Use the same techniques as for the public rooms, leaving on display only the items that are peaceful, beautiful, and useful. Store, recycle or toss the rest.

4. Clear out anything you hate

Take a look around the whole house and notice if there is anything you don't like the look or feel of. Desk you inherited from mean Uncle Charlie? Give it away; the bad vibes are bringing down the energy of the house. (The next owner will be able to appreciate it for itself, not having suffered old Uncle Charlie's bad temper or whatever is associated with that item.)

Make a few aesthetic upgrades, like finding a nice old crock or tin and stowing the dog food in it, rather than see the ugly bag on your kitchen floor.

5. Clear out anything that is broken

Anything that can't be quickly fixed or that is not worth fixing has got to go. Now is your chance to get out from under a few items that have languished on your "to do" list. Take your antique clock to the repairman, toss out the ice crusher with the frayed cord—you have had a crushed ice dispenser in your refrigerator door for five years now and don't need it! Clearing broken items will make room for functionality and set the tone for health improvements.

6. Clear out unsightly and dysfunctional items

Scan your home for the unsightly things you have gotten used to, like tangles of wires under the TV, and tie them up together after sorting them out. Replace trash cans that are too small and are constantly overflowing. Rearrange items your loved one needs close at hand so they are more easily reached.

7. Basements and attics—a special challenge

Frank Lloyd Wright refused to put basements or attics in his home designs because he felt it just encouraged collections of useless items. When tackling an area that stores seldom or never-used items, try this system: first, go through clutter and systematically remove things you want to keep using these criteria:

> Pull out:
>
> - Things that are useful, on a monthly, seasonal or yearly basis, such as Christmas decorations. Sort through these for broken, ugly, never used, and duplicate items and take only the good bits.
> - Things of great sentimental value; take only things you actually like and want to look at every now and then. Pare down that crate of kids' drawings to a nice sampler that fits in one small box or album.
> - Keep things that are beautiful, really beautiful.

8. What to do with the "keep pile"

You should have only a small "keeper" pile. Sort random objects into your seasonal bins, to be pulled out and put on display on a rotating basis. Bigger collections, like Christmas decorations, can be sorted into stackable bins with labels on the end. Don't make the bins too big or heavy or you might be tempted to leave them right where they are!

doctor's office should any other problems arise during Mom's stay. Better still, it was only twenty minutes from my brother's house. Insurance paid for everything here and we had only to fill out the requisite forms to authorize payment for Mom's new home for the next three months.

My brother and I felt like astronauts who had just completed a complicated moon mission. We had gotten our mother the best, most cheerful environment with the best food and nurses and doctors within five days of her fall. For the next 100 days, she would be set. For a change, we were in complete agreement about how best to care for Mom and she really appreciated that. When we fussed with each other about her care, it troubled her and she asked us repeatedly to please get along. It was nice to feel the glow of a job well done as a team for a change.

It was a big surprise to me that Mom would not ride to her new home in an ambulance. They just gave her an extra dose of painkillers and packed her carefully into the front seat of the big cushy car my brother rented for the ride. They said she would not be too uncomfortable on the 100-mile journey north to the Goodwin House, and we had no choice but to believe them. I checked in by cell phone with my brother as I followed along in my small SUV.

When we pulled up in the long circular driveway of the Goodwin House, an aide came out and helped Mom from the car and into a wheelchair. The hip was not a problem, but the cut on her leg was a worry. It had been carefully bandaged that morning for the trip and we asked that it be elevated as we made our way to the nursing floor. We made quite a procession. I had lent Mom one of my long black skirts that morning as she had only pants with her and did not think she could fit them over her bandages. With her leg stuck out in front with its furry bed sock poking out from the scalloped hem of my black linen skirt and my brother and I trailing behind with the luggage, including vases of flowers, bags of books and chocolates she had collected from well wishers at the hospital, we crammed into the small elevator and up to Mom's room.

Even at this excellent facility, there were no single rooms. Mom had a roommate who was dressed and sitting up in her bed when we arrived. She simply sat, propped up with pillows, eyes open, staring straight ahead never responding to any of our friendly "hellos." From time to time, she muttered softly. At night, an orderly sat in a chair by the door because she got up and wandered out sometimes. During Mom's entire stay, she never spoke to any of us, Mom included. I never once saw a visitor with her. Sad.

Mom's new room was bright and furnished with "antiques" that looked a bit like they had been culled from what residents had left behind when they moved on. But the sunshine and view from the broad windows was lovely and there was a curtain dividing her half of the small room from her silent roommate's bed, so mom could have privacy. In the hallways, my nose detected the faint scent of urine and disinfectant, fighting with the scent of old money. I fought the nausea and anxiety that rose up in my throat at the thought of leaving my mother here. Feeling I would never be able to stay in a place like this, I tried to stuff my feelings down beneath a front of good cheer and optimism.

Luckily, Mom was so disoriented with painkillers and residue of anesthesia that it did not seem to affect her the same way. From her standpoint, a hospital bed, a wheelchair, and a round-the-clock staff to help her might have seemed a bit more important than the fact that to get to the bathroom she had to skirt the bed of her zombie like roommate.

We unpacked Mom's few possessions and helped her figure out the controls to her bed and the small TV that was on the dresser, a bit too small far away for her entertainment, given the state of her eyesight now. Again, I counted us lucky she got the bed by the window as I placed her plants and vases and get-well cards there for her to appreciate. There was a dining room down the hall and we wheeled Mom down for dinner, bandaged leg poking out from the big black skirt. After some confusion about reserved tables (apparently there was some system of seniority in the dining room), we were hustled into a smaller and more elegant room and given menus. The selections were not broad, but the offerings sounded tasty and, indeed, the food was excellent. After dinner we got Mom settled back in bed and promised to return next the day. I could tell she was scared and tired, but the staff insisted we leave and that she would be fine.

And she was. Mom's mind was perfectly intact under all the meds and all it took was a few days for her to scope out the entire staff. She soon charmed the ones who needed to be charmed and stayed out of the way of the rest. When I visited, she liked to point out who was "tough as nails" and who was "nice as pie." My brother and I could not have been happier to see her emerging from the fog of painkillers and engaging in something other than her own drama. She even started reading books on her Kindle.

Soon she knew the story of everyone on the floor and loved telling us all the gossip. She made friends with one resident who had come to the nursing floor to recover from a fall. Her husband, who had lived with her in their independent apartment on twelfth floor until he got Alzheimer's, now lived in the "Hope Garden" floor of the facility, but joined her for dinner every evening. He was charming but vague and greeted us warmly several times during the meal, introducing himself politely every time and asking our names, where we came from, etc. The repetitive conversation was a challenge, but we soon got used to dining with this cheerful couple.

My mother loves to dress with flair, so my niece and I bought her new outfits that were better suited to her new slim shape and managing the transitions, bed to walker, walker to toilet, dressing and undressing. Loose, soft drawstring pants were deemed the best with long-sleeved, light-weight shirts or jackets. Mom had taken a liking to my shawls and I made sure she had a few cheerful ones to dress up her outfits and fight off the AC chill. For me, the highlight was seeing her proudly demonstrating her growing expertise with her walker as she steered us away from the dinner selections that she had found "not up to snuff" in the dining room cafeteria line which she had graduated to.

My brother and I heaved a huge collective sigh of relief. There is nothing sweeter than knowing that your ailing mother is being well-cared for in a safe, cheerful place and that she was applying herself to the mission of healing.

I drove back to New Hampshire checked in on my former life. Amazingly enough it was still there waiting for me. I visited my office, caught up with the latest clients and projects, and stopped by my New York property on the way to and from Virginia. The drive was now a mere ten hours and that made the trip so much easier for me. I don't mind long drives and used the time to catch up with business and friends on the cell phone (hands free) and listen to recorded books.

I tried to get down every two to three weeks and called Mom in between. My brother had a full house, so I often stayed in a hotel near the rehab center. Sometimes I flew down for just the day and flew back the same night. This was not as easy as it sounds because I live two hours from the airport, but if I left early enough in the morning; it was manageable. Knowing that Mom was safe, relatively happy, working hard on her own rehabilitation, and eating well to build up her strength and health was a wonderful feeling, but it couldn't go on forever.

It was time to think about the next move. Could she return to her home? Not without some major changes. My brother had begun a full renovation of Mom's home while she was away. We had decided that the updates she would need would also make the house more salable and be a good investment if we decided to go that way. Keeping our options open seemed the best plan. Even with the renovation, we realized that staying there on her own would not be a great idea. It would put us back where we began, with Mom isolated from society, and subject to another fall. We had gotten used to the relative convenience of seeing Mom in Northern Virginia and hated to think of the long, long road back "down home." We doubted she would drive again (a big relief all around), and that alone would have made life back home a challenge, as she would be dependent upon her home health aides for everything. They would need to come every day, which would be costly.

I had explored the option of relatively independent living in an elder community and learned that people live longer, some say six years on average, when they are part of a community with all the support services they need close at hand. Whether it was the better nutrition from having your meals prepared for you, the socialization of a community of your peers, or having medical professionals nearby, I could not say, but the evidence was compelling. Compared to a housebound life, it looked very attractive.

Maybe the smartest thing would be to fix up her house to sell. With the money from selling her house, we could perhaps find a place for Mom where she could be well looked after—if only for a year or so until she was really on her feet again. We knew Mom would fight us, but moving back to her old house was not the answer for now. In any case, the renovations were not near completion by the time Mom would be done with rehab. We decided that we would pitch this new move as "transitional," and maybe it would be. Looking back, I am pretty sure both my brother and I knew this would be permanent. If Mom truly hated it, we could always move her back home, and I would be staying there a lot.

Hunting for Home

Once my brother and I realized that a new place was in order, we started on yet another mission, this time to look at nearby elderly communities. We wanted one that offered all three levels of care: independent living apartments, assisted-living studios, and full-time nursing care, because we never wanted to have to go through this uprooting again. If we found just the right place, everyone could relax a bit and go back to appreciating each other rather than constantly worrying about "what next?"

To qualify for most places that offered all three levels of care, one first has to be healthy enough for independent living. By the time mom left rehab in three months, she would make the grade. It is usually okay if you need some help to keep you there, such as a home health aide.

Our goal was to find a place that would win mom over and inspire her to keep up her exercise, her nutrition, and give her more good years. We hoped she would like it, but we were prepared to live with a little grumbling if that's what it took.

First, we looked at the Goodwin House where she was now living on the nursing care floor. They had a number of empty apartments available in their independent-living section. While the Goodwin House was highly regarded, it had a complicated "buy-in" scheme. You could not rent; you had to buy and the price for the independent-living apartments was pretty steep to my mind. Moreover, there was a hefty monthly service fee that varied according to the "value" of the apartment you chose. But we soon learned that the purchase price of your apartment was non-refundable; you could not sell nor leave it to your heirs. The Goodwin House looked upon the purchase price as something of a donation to the nonprofit faith-based organization affiliated with the Episcopal church that ran it.

The monthly service fee went to operating costs and included one meal a day, some housekeeping services, and all the elder activities sit and fit in a piece or two. The furnishings were comfortable with fresh upholstery set in conversation groupings reminiscent of a grand hotel. This pleasant, light-filled space smelled of sunshine and care.

We looked at the apartments on the nursing and continuing care floor and found them to be cheerful and spacious. Should mom need more care, even temporarily, this would be an option right in the building.

Then we looked at the independent living options from one bedroom to large two-bedroom residences with den and balcony. Each apartment came with call buttons built in, in case one needed help, as well as a clip or necklace button that was tied to the 24/7 security office. Each apartment had a lock and a key. The entry to the building for non-residents was screened in the first floor lobby by a kind and cheerful receptionist named Hattie. She was not a resident but lived nearby and still drove herself to work everyday. Hattie retired shortly after Mom moved in having worked well into her nineties!

Attached outside each apartment door was a discrete little piece of Formica that was propped up vertically every night by the security staff. When the door is opened each morning, it flips down, letting the next security round know the resident is out and about. If the tag is not down, the resident is contacted to see if they require assistance.

To our delight, we found apartments that were as big as a house! The ceilings were high, the heat and air conditioning worked well, and the hallways were nicely furnished, well lit, and welcoming. Because the Jefferson had twenty-two floors of apartments in two towers, each floor was of a manageable size, giving this rather large facility a cozy feel.

We were invited to lunch and found that although most residents saved their one meal a day, which came along with the maintenance fee, for dinner, a lively group of healthy looking seniors were all dressed up and enjoying their lunch. The food was tasty and we got a look at the dinner menu for the week and saw with approval that residents could store their own personal wine collection in the wine cellar and be served their own vintages at dinner. House wine by the glass was also available.

Every Sunday, there was a festive Champagne Brunch. This feature quickly became one of our favorites for family gatherings. With reservations, residents may invite as many friends and family they liked for a small extra fee per person. All three meals—breakfast, lunch, and dinner—could be enjoyed in the dining room or delivered to one's apartment if desired. This would solve Mom's nutritional needs for sure.

There were a variety of sizes and prices for apartments. Best of all, we could rent or buy, and we decided renting was our best plan for now. What did it cost to secure this special place for my mom? Not as much as the other places we had looked at, especially considering we had no long-term commitment or up front buy in costs. The service fees were hefty, but then that was the case with all the residences we looked at. The Jefferson let you purchase your apartment outright with full rights, so you could sell it on your own or leave it your heirs. Prices ranged from $79,000 up to $395,000, depending on size. The service fees added an additional monthly cost from $2,000 to $4,000 per month and were based on square footage and the number of people living in each apartment.

They had about twenty apartments available for rent or sale at that time. None of the other places we looked at offered such a good choice of rentals. I worried there was something I was not seeing in this too-good-to-be-true place, but as we learned this glut of apartments was due to the fact that The Jefferson had opened thirty years ago when the concept of luxury senior residences was new. The value was so great that they quickly sold all the apartments in the building. At that time most of the purchasers were in their sixties and had now lived out their lives happily at The Jefferson. These apartments were all hitting the market just as the economy took a nose dive.

Here is a list of your possibilities:

Option One: Aging in Place

If aging at home is what you have decided upon, there are many agencies that will send in home health aides, nurses, housekeepers, etc., to support aging relatives. More than 7.5 million Americans currently receive home care, and there are more than 17,000 agencies that provide a variety of services.

Skilled nursing is available in the home for things like postoperative care, wound care, drug therapy, and cardiovascular disease management. Health aides can provide assistance with basic needs like dressing, eating, bathing, and toileting. Homemakers are available for grocery shopping, cooking, cleaning, and laundry. Depending on a senior's needs, physical, occupational, and speech therapists are also available.

Option Two: Retirement Communities

There are many styles and flavors of retirement communities. You need to tour the ones in your area to get a feel for the services offered. The costs for these and the financial structure vary widely.

Many offer cultural, social, and recreational opportunities that enrich the lives of the residents, creating an inviting environment that is far more stimulating than staying at home. They usually offer one to three meals a day (so nutritional needs may be easily met), most offer exercise classes, library, and transportation to stores, church, and social events as well as to doctor appointments.

One big benefit of these communities is that the residents are fully independent, while having their support services right on site. A call button for assistance will bring someone to the apartment in a few minutes; there is a daily check to see if the resident has left the apartment; there are on site nurses, podiatrists, and drivers to make life simple and safe again.

The residents of these communities I have spoken to were almost all reluctant to move in, but were later sorry they had not made the move sooner.

Option Three: Assisted-Living Facilities

This type of facility offers more support with meals, housekeeping, and help with other activities of daily living, like bathing and dressing. The resident spaces are usually smaller, with limited kitchen facilities. Staff will help administer and monitor medication.

Elderly housing in this category will often offer amenities like a fitness center or pool, but additionally provide options like onsite physical therapists, scheduled outings, spa treatments, and in-house hair salons. These services are usually a la carte, and you will generally pay for things like personal trainers, parking spaces, spa treatments, and haircuts.

Some assisted-living facilities have a special wing for Alzheimer's patients offering more monitoring of movement and cognitive therapy. The assisted-living wing is often a part of a larger retirement community offering three levels of assistance including the independent living apartments and nursing home.

Option Four: Nursing Homes

If a temporary setback like major illness or surgery mandates significant medical care and twenty-four-hour nursing supervision, the expertise and staffing levels of a nursing home may be required. A different elderly housing situation may be more appropriate down the line, but as a bridge between hospital care and a return to independent living, nursing homes can provide intensive rehabilitation services that other elderly housing cannot. These facilities can also be the best option when medical and nursing care will be required long term.

those rides. Not having a grandmother of their own, they started calling her Granny and were happy to spend time with her. She taught them to cut out sewing patterns and quilt piecing. They were thrilled. She gave them advice and *tsk-tsked* at them for choices they were making in their lives..

One of these women eventually became a nurse's aide and provided a lot of care for my mother in her last few months. My sister and I had several people lined up to care for Mom when we could not, or by our choice, would not do her personal care. Eventually, she needed someone to be with her at all times.

Nonetheless Mom managed to live independently up until the last three months of her life. She lived across the street from me for ten years, in an apartment that was set up for wheelchair access, which she needed for her last four years. Hot and stuffy, there was small kitchen with an open living and dining area where she had her favorite pieces of furniture. Her custom-made, black walnut round table with the base made from an antique iron sewing machine, foot pedal and all, sat with the antique-caned chairs and her Danish modern furniture that she loved. Shades of purple, turquoise, and brown created a serene room with pictures of her family, her china, her collection of antique irons and modern paintings everywhere.

The sheer drapes on the glass doors leading out to her deck overlooking the river filtered sunlight onto her collection of plants that seemed to wither along with her. Sometimes she would ask me to water them, offering her criticism and advice while I attempted to revive them, the water running through the weak soil. If I brought her a new plant she would sigh and say, "What do I need that for?" While I made room for the new plant, I would retort, "It's alive, Mom."

One corner of her apartment was devoted to her sewing table, with an adjacent closet filled with fabric in plastic drawer units separated by type and color, and enough sewing notions to start a store. There were boxes filled with every piece of clothing that had meaning to her, things she made for herself and for us as children. Things I thought I had thrown away would come back to be worn by grandchildren or recycled into a quilt. Calicos had been cut into triangles waiting to be made into her special potholders, which everyone loved getting at Christmastime.

It was her couch that always surprised everyone. Appearing uncomfortable, the couch I had known since I was five years old had scratchy, turquoise wool upholstery. It was eight feet long with soft cushions despite their itchiness that made that sofa the best place for napping. It would invite me to lie down, and within minutes I would be fast asleep. I would wake and Mom would still be at her table reading the paper or playing solitaire, and she would say, "I guess you were tired; overdoing it again." Another *tsk* and "You do too much, you need more sleep." When we had to stay overnight, it was the only place to sleep in her small apartment. The helpers that stayed with her didn't seem to mind, but I started to resent that couch. I would fight with myself about sitting on it because I knew it would soon draw me down to sleep, to escape the boredom of caregiving, the reality of my life—busy, too busy for sleep.

My mother loved to knit, and her knitting projects (socks, mittens, hats) along with balls of yarn were stuffed into plastic bags surrounding her bedroom. I had arranged her room to offer her easy access to all she needed when she was alone, everything within arm's reach. She even had a system of strings attached to pull chains for moving items around. The best things ever invented are those long-handled claw devices, which she frequently used for picking things up off the floor.

Sometimes when I went to her apartment to see her after my workday, she would be propped up in bed, reading a book, usually a mystery, with a stack of read and unread books waiting nearby. Dropping other and took turns keeping Mom company, sitting at her bedside.

Mom kept her dry sense of humor those last days saying to my brother, "Behave yourself." He responded, "We will," and she replied, "That's no fun!" Before she drifted off, she said, "Everybody's here and here I am, the crabby old bitch!"

To me she said, "I wanted to wait to the end of March to die, but I don't think I can—or was it the end of January, but . . ." and then her voice faded away. I told her I was here and she looked at me and said, "You're a sweetheart." That was the last thing she said to me and it may be the best thing I ever heard from her.

About forty-eight hours before she died, Mom began her "life review," as the hospice nurse called it. She stopped talking to us directly and her eyes stayed closed while her mind went wherever she took it. Muttering to herself almost non-stop she uttered words in random order. She mentioned so many things, places she lived, people she knew, our family dog, she seemed to be putting them all into safe keeping in her mind to carry with her to wherever she was going.

Eventually, she stopped talking but I could see her mind was still working; despite her eyes being closed, I could see rapid-eye movement. What was amazing was seeing her hands moving around in front of her face and over her hair, as if she was trying to put in the clear plastic hair combs that she always wore. Her hands seemed to be recalling all her memories.

In the end Mom's journey to the other side lasted only two days and her breathing slowed gradually. In the end, it really does come down to something as simple as the breath. We kept watching her breathing, expecting her to take one more breath, or expecting her to stop, and then she did, calmly taking in her last breath. She died surrounded by most of her family. My brother, his wife, my son, my grandson, niece and a friend were present and we cried together, hugged, and said good-bye to this powerful woman who was our mother, grandmother, great-grandmother. As my niece, Piper, put it "I think there was no more peaceful way for Grandma to go. She was surrounded by family, surrounded by her pictures and things, and had the quiet of Tracey's home. Once she stopped fighting, she just slipped away; quietly we all stood around her holding hands."

Moving Beyond

Calling the hospice nurse at three in the morning felt a bit intrusive, but she said, "Like birth, death is unpredictable; I am on call, you call me when you need me." So I called. She was a lovely woman with a nice accent and peaceful countenance, and she arrived quickly as promised after Mom died. She and I washed Mom's body, dressing her in her favorite flannel night gown and a pair of her hand-knit socks. She would have hated it if we had put her in fancy clothes. "What a waste," she would say. She probably would have preferred that I give the socks to one of the grandchildren, but I wanted her to feel cozy.

Brushing her hair, placing her hair combs carefully, I broke down, sobbed, realizing this would be the last time she needed me to do her hair for her and that was it. All of the children and grandchildren that were present came in and said good-bye to her one more time. She was ready for cremation. The Cremation Society came later that morning and took her body away.

To this day, whenever I see plastic hair combs, I think of Mom's beautiful thick hair, how she finally let it go white, and how even as she died, it seemed that she wanted her combs in place.

"Afterwards we all went back into the living room and after a little silence, the memories started flowing. We all traded favorites and laughter began to replace tears. I remembered food—Grandma will always be associated with gingersnaps, Triscuits, and Wise Pride cheese spread. Oh, and ginger ale! Crossword puzzles, of course, and all her great stories. Her irons, her necklaces, and her sending of birthday cards and checks. We remembered her with love and she will be missed." *Written in the journal we kept at my mother's bedside by my niece, Piper Goodeve, February 27, 2009*

"I do not fear death. I had been dead for billions and billions of years before I was born, and had not suffered the slightest inconvenience from it."

Mark Twain

Tracey Interviews A Geriatric Medicine Specialist

Dr. Leo Cooney of Yale University has spent the past forty years of his medical career working on issues related to the care of the elderly. On a warm spring day, he shared his experience and knowledge with me. Exuding patience and care with an obvious gentle demeanor, a peaceful countenance and a broad smile, he was generous with his time and highlighted the many issues facing us all as we age.

"As you age, you collect chronic conditions, so your chance of getting chronic conditions increases. So at fifty, your risk is zero, at sixty-five your risk is three conditions, at eighty it's five conditions. I think the major things that produce decline in older people are dementia, chronic disabling conditions, medical conditions, falls, arthritis, you can try to prevent these things as much as possible by staying physically and intellectually fit; try to avoid diabetes, try to avoid falls, you can do all of that, but the key to living an old age, that is after about eighty-five, is adapting."

This adapting to change is a hard thing, for everyone. Learning to live with a body that is growing older every day in a society that has told us repeatedly that we are 'less than' because of our age leaves us open to depression and a rapid decline if we give up hope. Dr. Cooney stressed the importance of self-esteem and contentment in old age.

"First and foremost, what we talk about here is try to focus on the contentment of the old person, because I see of lot of conflict between caregivers and the people being cared for. A lot of that is because these fifty-year-old daughters think their eighty-year-old mother should change her diet, increase her exercise and, I'm not saying it's not good to do those kind of things, but I think the bottom line is that what's important to elderly people is how they feel about themselves and how contented they are. That's really the Holy Grail at any point in life.

mother, I would raise her pillow by pillow up to the step stool then use more pillows to help catapult her into bed. Her arms were strong from years of wheelchair use, so she could help me a lot.

Then once I got her settled onto the bed, I would have to help her with whatever she was doing when she fell, either getting dressed or undressed, getting into bed or into her wheelchair, going to or from the bathroom. Often it turned into a full bath and dressing routine and I would return home hours later.

One day she called to tell me that she was sitting on the ground in the parking lot outside her house where she had fallen while getting into her friend's car. She had a nervous laugh and said, "I didn't really fall; I just slid down the edge of the car seat to the ground," as she was transferring into the car from her wheelchair while her elderly friend tried to help but mostly stood by helplessly watching. Luckily, I was home and again I ran across the street and when I got there, Mom smiled up at me with her sardonic laugh saying, "I'm okay; I just can't get up!" They were both somewhat shaken by this incident, her friend more so than Mom.

What astounded me was that Mom would take all this with her sense of humor and a certain amount of ease and childlike hopefulness. Her attitude was this very haphazard "gee-I-hope-Tracey-is-there," kind of thing. Once I was at work when she called for help and I could not get there. Luckily, I was able to get a friend to go help her back into bed; otherwise, an ambulance would have to have been summoned. Luckily, she never broke any bones and managed to avoid years of nursing home care! Most of the time I was there for her because I knew I had to be, often resenting having to live by this unwritten plan of hers.

Tracey's Hope For Her Future

This is exactly what I want to avoid with my own children. Like Mary, I do not expect my children to care for me unless they want to; which is not to say that I do not want to be close to them as I grow older. I want to see their lives unfold, to see my grandchildren grow up and create a whole new world for themselves. I want to be in their lives. Is there a way to do this without making them have to manage my probable need for some sort of caretaking? I hope that I am healthy and strong until my dying day, but I am also a realist. If I do need care at some distant, future point, I have my long-term care insurance in place.

I am working on my plan on how to age without being "a burden" be it physically, financially, but most especially, emotionally. I want my children to feel free to decide how they want to live their lives without worrying about me. My hope is to find a way to keep stimulated; to keep growing mentally, intellectually; to keep active; to continue to live independently as I grow older; to have choices.

Here is a great quote from a high-school friend: "It's not that we are old; it's that we were so young!" Looking at pictures of her with her smooth skin, brown hair, an eagerness and openness evident in her face, life seemed so endless then. We were young in heart, mind, and body.

Time travel to forty-five years later. We have been married, divorced, married again, raised children, taken care of elderly or ill parents, held their hands while they died. All the while negotiating our work life so we could take care of others in need.

Now when we are together; we are the same fifteen-year-old girls we used to be. We look forward to more new adventures; they might just be a little different than they were forty years ago! Family, home, parents, work; this is the stuff life is made of.

How do we keep living while we are growing old or up? (I have friends who are still asking themselves what they want to do at age sixty-two!) Some are "done" with their lifelong work and long for something different. Making a change in career or lifestyle can be a daunting task at age fifty-five or sixty. But why not? Colonel Harland Sanders of Kentucky Fried Chicken began his career in fast food at the age of sixty-five! All the latest research shows that baby boomers will not want to retire at sixty-five. For lots of reasons—financial, emotional, intellectual—most intend to keep working well into their eighties.

Aging does not necessarily mean giving up one's independence. It may mean that independence is defined differently, that we become interdependent in new ways. What is hard to avoid is the idea that we may become victims of our age. Feeling worthless or less valued because we can no longer do the things that gave our lives meaning. Finding the right place to live out one's remaining years is vitally important because it will impact our health and well-being. Looking at another thirty to forty years of life, what do you want to do?

The world has gotten much more accessible. It is easier to get around, to travel. Opportunities for personal growth and adventures are everywhere. Sit home and read? Maybe. Zip line through the canopy in Costa Rica? How old is too old to be doing that? Will my body sustain itself through the world of adventures out there in the big world? I sure hope so; I have a lot of things I would like to do.

Looking Good/Feeling Well

As my eighty-seven-year-old father has been telling me for years, "You have to keep moving." He is living proof that exercise works wonders. He walks on the treadmill, lifts weights, rides the bicycles, or swims. He likes to say, "I wake up in the morning, I get out of bed, and put one foot in front of the other and keep going until I've gone to the gym and I'm home again."

In the months following his knee surgery, I would often hear him say to me, "You look tired." "I am," I reply. *Could be because I am worried about you*, I say to myself. Tired from working full time, plus some, taking care of children, grandchildren, myself, and you!

Does he think I look tired or just old? "I'm fifty-six years old," I tell him. He looks at me wide-eyed as if he can't believe it. I think, yes, I'm not fourteen anymore, though sometimes I feel like it. I still want to have fun; I want to be free to do as I please. I want to go horseback riding. Last year Dad told me he wanted to ride a horse, something he always wanted to do but hadn't done since he was a kid. Maybe this year I will take him. We could go together.

I took lessons as a kid but haven't been on a horse since about twenty-two years old. I would love to go to where the wild horses roam, to see them running free. Lately, I've been thinking about taking my grandchildren to a dude ranch out west. Is this something a grandmother does with her grandchildren? Why not? I want to. I want to be strong enough and healthy enough to ride, too.

I have stayed strong by keeping active. I look at people I know who are my age or younger and I see the results of a sedentary life. A body old before its time. I want to wander the streets of Paris someday with my granddaughter. In ten years, I will be sixty-six and she will be thirteen—a perfect time to take her to Paris. A treat for me and for her, to create a good memory for her to remember her old grandmother. This and so much more I have to look forward to as I become an old woman. I have to stay strong and healthy by taking care of myself for my children's children.

Dad still wants to go horseback riding. "Let's do it this spring," I tell him, "Funny you say that, I've been looking at the horse farm down the road." "Okay, Dad, find out about it and we will do it." Now that he has a new knee, he should be able to ride. My sister is afraid that the reason he wants to ride a horse is so he can get one and ride it into town when he has to stop driving!

Tracey's Top Ten Tips for Acting Your Age

Every magazine I pick up lately has articles about "aging gracefully." They have photos of thirty or forty-year-olds with *a* wrinkle or *one* gray hair. The advice is all about tips focusing on how to "not look old" or "stay looking younger longer." There are the latest tricks for hair and makeup for women and hints for men to stay virile and strong. It may be a nice premise but they hold a lot of vain promises and I find myself getting agitated, because I think graceful aging is more than looking "not-old." Graceful aging is about having increased patience and charm, wisdom and grace. Knowing when to open your mouth and roar like a lion or when to keep quiet. These traits can only be acquired with age and experience.

1. **Count your successes!** Keep your diplomas, certificates, awards where you see them every day, even if it was some silly ribbon you won in high school.

2. **Be generous** with yourself and your possessions.

3. **Start a memory book** for your children's children. Write down your story, or tell it into a tape recorder.

4. **Get outside** every day, we all need fresh air and sunshine, no matter how young or old you are!

5. **Practice yoga**, or some kind of balancing/stretching movement like tai chi. Stretch your muscles and tendons every day, this helps to strengthen your bones and prevent falls.

6. **Get your papers in order.** Keep a list of where you have your important papers; give a copy to a trusted child, friend, or lawyer.

7. **Let your family know** what your plans are for your old age before it gets here. Draw up a living will, you can download one from the internet and have it notarized.

8. **Listen to your body**. If you have pain, pay attention to what your body is telling you. Seek medical advice.

9. **Seek alternative body work.** Consider anything that helps you to feel better and does not cause more harm. That includes pedicures, manicures, steam rooms, saunas, hot tubs, massage therapists, chiropractic care, physical therapists, acupuncture. Do get medical care for illnesses that do not respond to your self-care or alternative therapies.

10. **Consider all medical advice** to be just that—advice. You can take it or leave it. Do you really want to spend your remaining time in the hospital on chemotherapy? Or do you want to go on that cruise you have put off, or rent that beach house you have wanted to do since you were in college?

11. **Be happy.** Do what gives you pleasure; share your happiness.

Mary Boone's Dream of Blue Sky Aging

I once spent a summer at an ashram, meditating and taking courses on spiritual betterment. My friends said, *How nice for you to have such a lovely retreat*, but I said, "Retreat, that was no retreat; it was an advance!" I felt I was charging onward, ever onward into my life, as I deepened my spiritual side.

One of the courses offered that summer was called the "No Ego" course. It was restricted to students under the age of fifty. The older population of the ashram politely rebelled, demanding to know why they could not better themselves by reducing their egos, too? The answer came down from the guru that people over fifty should be contemplating their own deaths, not trying to diminish their ego. I guess if our ego survived fifty years, it was considered an asset. Maybe we needed it to take us through the later years while we contemplated our death!

Except that the thought that they would even consider dying was a big shock to that older crowd. It seemed somehow impolite to point out the finite nature of life. To some, it was a wake-up call to buckle down and start practicing the highflying principles we had been discussing all summer; to others it was a challenge to their sense of self as vital and useful members of society.

I was in my forties at the time and was not too concerned with the issue, but it comes to mind today at the age of sixty-two as I am on the brink of a "maturity" that undeniably falls in the second half of life.

There has been a slow but profound shift in my mindset about aging and death. I realize finally that I really am coming up against the deadline of all deadlines. I know that eventually the "pencils down" call will come and the test of my life will be over. I will have done what I had the strength, will, and love to do. I will have made my contribution through a thousand small nudges toward the reality we all inhabit, and I can hope that I improved that reality a little bit. Regardless, I will have no choice but to move on. At the very least, I will be able to say I have tasted some of life's great and glorious vintages and I have enjoyed them without reservation.

While I may have no sway over how or when I will go, I do have the power to make good choices about how I will age. I have the power to make choices that keep me strong and prepare me for a healthier future. I have the power to choose the right nutrition, I have the power to work my body hard, but with respect, so it will be strong and flexible enough to carry me through to the end. I have the power to share what I know and what gives me joy, so I can stay connected to the people and the world I love.

I have wonderful pictures of my future in my mind, places to go and people to spend time with, vintages to sample. Whether the cruises I take are on an ocean-going yacht with caviar and champagne, or the plank with a sail pinned to a broom for a mast out in my backyard where I eat peanut butter and jelly sandwiches with my grandchildren—the trips are just as real, just as meaningful. I plan on sailing into my future with more enthusiasm, less fear, and as much fun as I can stir up for the rest of my life.

Mary Boone's Top Ten Tips for a Long Life

I have been collecting ideas for flourishing health and long life as long as I can remember. Here are my current favorites. Only the most delicious and delightful recommendations have made my list. By the way, they are all scientifically proven to be of benefit, so you really can't go wrong.

1. **Drink** - It makes you merry—but only one glass. Red wine has antioxidants that sharpen the mind and slow aging. If you drink too much, buy very expensive wine—that always slows me down! On weekends I have a glass of scotch for variety.

   Drink (Part Two) - Drink some more, but this time, drink water. Water keeps things moving, literally. (Note: If you like to drink a lot of coffee or tea, be careful. The caffeine depletes your electrolytes.) I also use a humidifier in the dry months. This outer hydration keeps your skin nice and plump.

2. **Eat chocolate** - Every day, but only the very, very good kind; darker the better. Indulge in imported, organic chocolate or whatever floats your boat.

3. **Keep learning and stay relevant** - Keep up to date with technology. Add a new computer skill each week. Call the helpline if you get stuck. It is important to stay current. Read the newspaper and magazines—you can get them online and adjust the type size, so there are no excuses. Keep up with your favorite public figures and current events. Research your next vacation, latest medical breakthroughs, and then share your new info with a friend.

4. **Keep in touch** - Skype, Twitter, send texts and emails to your young relatives, then plan to get together. You will be the coolest old person on the block! Establish connections with your friends and families and take it farther than a Facebook page. Plan a get-together! Make new friends who share your latest enthusiasms, worldview, and spiritual outlook.

5. **Laugh** - Watch a funny movie you have always loved; even better if you share it with someone. There is medical evidence that the very act of smiling triggers endorphins and serotonin, making us even-tempered and full of joy. You can download movies from several websites: www.hulu. com or www.netflix.com are two sites that let you download movies to your computer for a nominal fee. I love the BBC sense of humor! I once cured someone from a severe bout of depression by showing him one funny movie a day.

6. **Cry** - If laughing is good for your health, so is a good cry. Releasing emotions, especially sad ones, is also just as health-enhancing. When you lose a loved one, have a good cry, and then talk to someone about your feelings of loss. Don't keep your sadness bottled up inside. Let it out. Be patient with yourself and your grief. It takes time to rebuild your world without a loved one.

7. **Dress Snappy** - It does not cost a penny to take a little care with your appearance. Tie a scarf in a new way, mix and match your favorite outfits. Put on a little lipstick, but only if you are a woman or a clown, or maybe a transvestite. (Hey, Eddie Izzard looks great in a short skirt! If you don't know Eddie Izzard, go online and google him. Very, very funny! [see tip Number 5].)

8. **Floss!** - This doesn't sound like fun, but use the mint floss; it is refreshing and how nice is it to have a sparkling smile? My dentist says you only have to floss the teeth you plan to keep.

9. **Cover up** - Don't get sunburn. Some people think sunscreen is toxic, but you don't need it if you stay out of the sun. A little goes a long way. Use bronzer or get a spray tan if you like, but don't sacrifice your skin for vanity.

10. **Move!** - Train, exercise, or just move every day in some way that intentionally puts your body to the test. Choose your movement to suit your temperament, but do it every day and for heaven's sake, choose something you love to do!

Financial Planning for Old Age

Mary Boone Interviews a Financial Planner

I spoke to Bob O'Hara, CPA/PFS, CExP, who advises small business owners about exit strategies and planning for their retirement.

I asked Bob, "What can you do now if you haven't made any retirement plans? Is it too late to make a plan that will make a difference?"

"Most people I talk to are not emotionally prepared to retire. Shifting your identity away from a profession that defined you is very hard if you have no other interests." These are the people who become depressed after they leave their job, they never really get interested in anything else and die soon after. If you wait till the day you retire to look around for something else to do, you might find yourself depressed.

"I advise my clients to take some time in the few years before retirement to explore their interests and begin to develop other possibilities. That way you can transition into a different life you are sure will prove rewarding to you. I encourage people to think about their vision of life, one that can be lived outside their business or profession. On the first day, everyone envisions it will be like a vacation, but how do you think you will feel about an idle life a year later? The people who have really lived into their new life in their imagination first are the ones who will be happy, fulfilled, and enjoying their freedom."

Bob has found that before you can pull the trigger on even the best retirement plan, you have to come to terms with the realities of how life will be in the years after your working career is behind you. He advises to "keep it simple." Your plans for accumulating wealth will be more successful if you focus more on making regular deposits than on fancy investments. Compound interests on your retirement savings mean your youngest years are the most fruitful of all your working years; never mind, the amounts you are putting away are most probably the smallest. These are the dollars that have longer to grow and multiply. If you begin to save for your later years right from the start of your working life and make the savings automatic, so you never actually see the money in your available cash account, you will painlessly accumulate an astonishing pile by the time you are ready to kick back.

If you are older and have spent your early years just keeping up, it is time now to get serious about saving for old age. If you are putting this off while you continue to support your grown children because they are "having a hard time making it in today's world," you may want to consider how they might feel if you come up short of cash in your later years. They may be still struggling to make ends meet and will have hoped you took care of your future needs back when you had the chance.

"People look at what they will have to live on when they retire, they get so upset they just refuse to think about it anymore!" Keep in mind that by the time you retire, many of your current expenses will be gone; that is, you will have paid down your mortgage, presumably finished expanding and improving the house, and own a good car. On the other hand, because of rising costs—taxes, utilities, medical care, and the fact that your life may be longer than you planned for—Bob is afraid there might be a whole generation of people who do not have enough of a plan in place.

To address this, Bob said: "It is important to look ahead at the upcoming financial realities, for yourself and your loved ones. Calculate what you really spend each month, minus the expenses that will have disappeared by the time you retire, such as dry-cleaning, commuting costs, etc.. If your income is a regular-fixed one, you can look over the resources available and make a quick calculation about how long those resources will last. If you are waiting for the sale of a business or property, for the economy to turn around or the next big client or sale to bail out your future, it can be scary to stop and stare those financial realities down. Do it anyway."

Planning for Small Business Owners

Bob told me that there are some special issues with small business owners and entrepreneurs, an area he has focused on for years now. Many small business owners are approaching retirement age along with their senior management team. They are planning to hire a younger replacement team to manage their business after they retire so they can keep drawing their dividends while the business continues. These business owners have made a mistake by failing to calculate the difference in the size of the boomer generation and the GenX'ers who are the natural candidates for this job. There are almost half as many of them as boomers, so it may be a challenge to find willing and qualified people to continue even the most successful business.

"If you have key people in their early forties, you can't afford to lose them because there is no one out there to take their place. These people are commanding high salaries by virtue of their scarcity. This is an issue that goes across the economy, worldwide," Bob said. This surprised me given the current underemployment. I think small business owners and workers alike may have to re-think our retirement age and work longer just to keep businesses afloat while a new team trains to take over.

Because of these realities, many people will choose to work long into their later years. I think that I will probably never really retire. I have so many interests and plans, many of them for money-generating businesses or inventions, but knowing as I do now that there is a lot of work involved in creating an overnight success, I am being far more conservative with what I have now. My plan is to secure what I have and keep building on it.

I asked Loren Carlson, chairman of CEO Roundtable (http://www.ceo-roundtable.com), a Boston-based forum that brings CEOs, presidents, and company owners together to exchange information, ideas and insights, what the very successful executives he works with think about retirement.

"As I look back on the sixteen years of leading the CEO Roundtable, it is clear that very few CEOs 'retire' to leisure. Indeed, the great majority could easily afford to retire but long before it was time to, they had dismissed the idea and were making plans for their next adventure—often their next company or an enlarged role and responsibility in a non-profit organization. They want to continue to take on challenges and make a difference in the world. I think that some anticipated spending more time with grandchildren but suddenly realize the grandchildren are now young adults and invested in their own naturally self-centered lives. I have never heard one CEO say they wanted to spend their time playing golf; usually they say, 'How much golf can you play and maintain your sanity?' Retirement villages are not filled with CEOs."

Getting Focused on Your Financial Plan

1. Gather all your financial data for a good look at current assets and liabilities.

2. Use website calculators for a fast look at your future.

   For facts about your Social Security payments, visit: www.socialsecurity.gov/

   Use the retirement calculator on the AARP site to get an idea about your own future prospects (http://www.aarp.org/work/retirement-planning/retirement_calculator).

   This one is helpful because it allows you to plug in a large—one hopes—lump sum you may be expecting from an inheritance, the sale of a business, or perhaps downsizing the family home or selling off vacation property. With this calculator, you can play around with your retirement age, prospects, and expenses and play a budget game with your future. Do not panic! This is just a tool. There is time to fix things!

3. Seek inspiration from real-life money gurus. Dave Ramsey (www.daveramsey.com/) is good for his straightforward approach to reality and inspiring stories about people just like you us who made it through.

   Another good resource is Suze Orman, who will answer your questions at her site: www.suzeorman.com

4. Call a professional, talk to your accountant, or your financial planner. Find a professional in your area at: www.napfa.org/ (National Association of Personal Financial Advisors).

   Get second and third opinions and always seek the advice of an independent expert, not someone who hopes to sell you stock, mutual funds, or another financial instrument. The money you spend on an expert will pay off in peace of mind in the end.

   There are different designations for financial planners, here are the two most common:

   The CPA/PFS (personal financial specialist) is a CPA with a combination of tax expertise and a comprehensive knowledge of financial planning. The PFS credential is awarded exclusively to AICPA members who have demonstrated considerable experience and expertise in financial planning. (www.aicpa.org/interestareas/personalfinancialplanning)

   The CFP (certified financial planner) designation is a professional certification for financial planners conferred by the Certified Financial Planner Board of Standards on an individual who has demonstrated a level of financial planning technical knowledge and expertise in financial planning. (www.cfp.net)

   To find a fee only Financial Advisor (someone who charges a fee for their advice, rather than a percentage) in your area you can use the website of the National Association of Personal Financial Advisors (www.napfa.org)

5. Start now! Pay down your debts, save a fund in a certificate of deposit for emergencies. Keep this in a different bank so you really have to think before you use it. Then you can use the cash you used to use for debt service to pay off your mortgage and then to put money away for retirement.

Remember, it is more important to move in the right direction and get excited about your progress than to act from desperation. That way you will be inspired to keep making good financial choices. It's having the courage to take that first step that will pay off.

Exercise: Move It or Lose It

Seniors stand to benefit more than any other age group from regular exercise. Like caring for your finances, it is not as important that you begin with the perfect program, but that you begin—right now. Regular, daily exercise yields health benefits, both long term and short. Setting aside time each day to exercise needs to be a lifelong habit that may be begun at any age. Consider yourself an athlete who is in training for the biggest race of all: your life. Improvements in blood pressure, neurocognitive function, osteoporosis, and cholesterol have been noted fairly quickly. Exercise is essential to build up core strength that aids in balance, preventing falls.

Regular physical activity lowers the risk of Alzheimer's disease and dementia, diabetes, obesity, heart disease, osteoporosis, and colon cancer, to name just a few. The American Cancer Society recommends a physically active lifestyle, along with an appropriate weight and healthful diet, to prevent recurrence, second primary cancers, and other chronic diseases. Studies have shown that exercise improves cardiovascular fitness, muscle strength, body composition, fatigue, anxiety, depression, self-esteem, happiness, and quality of life in cancer survivors.

Here is a list of what a regular exercise program will improve:

- **Arthritis Pain** – Exercise increases strength and flexibility, reduces joint pain, and helps combat fatigue.
- **Diabetes Prevention** – In one lifestyle intervention program that included moderate physical activity for at least 150 minutes per week, exercise was found to be more effective than medication in reducing the incidence of diabetes.
- **Immune Function** – During moderate exercise, immune cells circulate through the body more quickly and are better able to kill bacteria and viruses. After exercise ends, the immune system generally returns to normal within a few hours, but consistent, regular exercise

seems to make these changes a bit more long-lasting. A healthy, strong body fights off infection and sickness more easily.

- **Cardio-Respiratory and Cardiovascular Function** – Regular physical activity lowers risk of heart disease and high blood pressure and can increase your lung capacity, strengthening breathing muscles and improving airflow in and out of your lungs.

- **Bone Density/Osteoporosis** – Exercise protects against loss in bone mass. Better bone density will reduce the risk of osteoporosis and lowers risk of falling. Increases in bone density can be had in as little as twelve to twenty minutes of weight-bearing exercise, three days a week, dramatically reducing the loss of bone mass and susceptibility to fractures.

- **Gastrointestinal Function** – Regular exercise promotes the efficient elimination of waste and encourages digestive health.

Regular physical activity lowers risk of Alzheimer's disease and dementia, diabetes, obesity, heart disease, osteoporosis, and colon cancer, to name just a few. The American Cancer Society recommends a physically active lifestyle, along with an appropriate weight and healthful diet, to prevent recurrence, second primary cancers, and other chronic diseases. Studies have shown that exercise improves cardiovascular fitness, muscle strength, body composition, fatigue, anxiety, depression, self-esteem, happiness, and quality of life in cancer survivors.

In addition to these medical improvements, you can expect:

- **Better Sleep** – People who perform regular exercise sleep more easily and deeply at night.

- **Stress Relief and Contentment**– Social interaction is a known stress reliever. Joining a fitness class or gym is a great way of meeting new people or a ten-minute walk with a friend helps reduce stress. Exercise helps release endorphins which makes you feel more contented and happier.

- **Weight loss** – Regular activity reduces excess weight, especially if done in conjunction with a calorie-controlled diet. Exercise is vital to maintain weight loss.

- **Better Joints** – Building the muscles around joints helps stabilize them, which helps with flexibility and to prevent falls..

- **Improved Mood** – Physical activity stimulates various brain chemicals (endorphins) that may leave you feeling happier and more relaxed. You may also feel better about your appearance, when you exercise regularly you boost your confidence and improve your self-esteem.

- **More Energy** – Regular physical activity can improve your muscle strength and boost your endurance. And when your heart and lungs work more efficiently, you have more energy to go about your daily chores.

- **Increased Brain Power** - A new study by Canadian researchers shows that an exercise program featuring resistance training improves the cognitive functioning of older women, and improves it by a good and noticeable margin. Researchers from Vancouver Coastal Health and the University of British Columbia followed eighty-six senior women with mild cognitive impairment for a six-month study. The study, which was published in the April 23, 2012 issue of *Archives of Internal Medicine*, as reported by *Science Daily*: [In case you want to look up the entire article: http://www.sciencedaily.com/releases/2012/04/120423162403.htm]

The women, who were between the ages of sixty-five and seventy-five, were divided into two groups; one performed resistance training exercises (weight training) and the other did aerobic exercise. The groups exercised twice a week for six months in sessions that lasted about an hour. Both of these groups were tested regularly to assess the brain functions needed for independent living—paying attention, memory, problem solving, and executive decision-making. They were also analyzed for brain plasticity (new brain cell growth) with a functional MRI.

The results showed big improvement in decision-making and memory with an increase in brain plasticity in the group performing weight training exercise. These are the very things that begin to decline in the early stages of Alzheimer's disease! The aerobic training group did not show these results, but that does not dismiss the benefits to your overall health.

"Exercise is attractive as a prevention strategy for dementia as it is universally accessible and cost-effective," said Liu-Ambrose, the lead researcher. The impact of weight training on the brain was so positive that the research team made a video and posted it on YouTube. Go to http://www.youtube.com/watch?v=vG6sJm2d4oc to see it and begin your new weight training program.

With all these factors in favor of exercise, why don't more people get going and set up a regular routine? The two biggest reasons are fear and lack of time. Starting out may be difficult, because inactivity equals loss of muscle mass and endurance, and the early days and weeks of any new exercise regimen can be daunting. By starting small, even the most frail senior can reap the benefits of strength and well-being that come with exercise. If lack of time is your concern, think of the time you would lose if you broke your hip or wrist. The key is to exercise regularly and to begin slow.

Your physician can refer you to the most beneficial types of exercise to begin with, and sometimes a program of physical therapy is a good place to begin. See if you can get a referral to work on your most pressing physical challenges. There are so many resources available for elder exercise it can be hard to choose. Making a commitment to attend a class might be just the thing to get you into your routine.

Finally, some people claim exercise is boring. Try selecting a new sport: biking on a recumbent bike or the open road, or take up tennis or swimming. All have health benefits and can be done with groups to make them fun.

Here are some sites with resources for exercise programs. Check with your doctor before beginning a new program.

http://www.eldergym.com/

http://www.strongerseniors.com

http://www.aarp.org/videos.video-name=Fat-2-Fit-The-Quest-to-Find-Enjoyable-Exercise/

Dental Health

Dr. Dana Bartlett is a forward thinking dentist in a very rural part of New Hampshire. You can summarize his message in a few short words— "Keep your teeth!"

Dr. Bartlett believes the most important thing for people to know is that their teeth are designed to last a lifetime, no matter how long that turns out to be,

Some people think that it is inevitable that they will lose their teeth, notes Dr. Bartlett, and they seem to think all their worries and pain will be over once that happens. "Losing your teeth in your eighties is a horrendous procedure. Having teeth extracted and adapting to prosthetic teeth is painful. People should try to avoid that because people who keep their teeth live longer!" says Dr. Bartlett.

It has been said that losing your teeth will take ten years off your life. Chewing is not as easy and you reduce the efficiency of chewing your food by 85% with prosthetic teeth. You are asking a lot of the gastrointestinal system to take over for what the teeth should be doing— breaking down your food before it hits your stomach. They will not be able to chew well, the dentures are painful, they smell, they taste awful, and half the time patients don't even wear them. They also won't last a lifetime and will need to be replaced every ten years.

"When people stop taking care of their teeth in their fifties, they lose their teeth in their sixties; it happens pretty fast." Dr. Bartlett says that dentures are so much worse than people ever dream they will be. One big problem is bone loss. When teeth are extracted, the bone that supported the teeth slowly reabsorbs into the body. This results in so little bone left that over time, the dentures cannot find a good seat, resulting in even less chewing power and shortening life. Unless it has some reason to be there, the bone disappears.

Dr. Bartlett adds: "What we do now is to put in small implants to retain the bone—the implant seats into the dentures, for a better fit." The implant gives the bone a reason to be there, so there is less bone loss. Anyone with dentures now should check into getting these small implants sooner rather than later. If too much bone is lost, this won't work. A lot of people who have ill-fitting dentures set themselves up for chronic mouth trouble in later life.

It will serve you to be proactive and keep your teeth for the rest of your life. With modern dentistry, that is very possible to do! The number one cause of loss of teeth is periodontal disease, infection of the bone and gum around the teeth. The loss of that support is why people lose teeth, not cavities as most people suppose.

People have to be diligent about home care and make sure they avoid infection with regular checkups. It is increasingly difficult for older people to have good home care because of loss of manual dexterity, arthritis, low vision, etc.

"We ask our elderly patients to use a powered toothbrush because it often gives better results." Dr. Bartlett added "they make all the differently shaped brushes, flossing aids, etc., for people who find it a challenge. Our profession is always looking for ways to prolong the natural life of teeth because medicine keeps prolonging the life of people!"

Dr. Bartlett continues "Elderly people with some disabilities may need help to remove all the plaque. A lot of patients who have had excellent hygiene up until they go into a nursing home and then all the teeth that have been stable for the last seventy-five years go downhill in five years without careful attention. This is a good thing to check if you have a loved one in a care facility."

Some elderly people, unless they have a younger person setting up appointments, providing transportation and being sure they go, may not follow through with good dental care.

Dr. Bartlett says, "Yes, it seems they forget more easily. If I ask my senior citizens when the last time they were in my office, they will say, 'Oh, three months ago,' when in fact it was three years ago! The concept of time is different for the older brain!"

Then, there are a lot of complications for older dental patients. A lot of older patients have prosthetic joints and they must be pre-medicated before a cleaning. They sometimes forget to take the medication, ahead of time and then have to be rescheduled.

One big plus to modern dental care is that it is rarely painful. Another is that, as old filings need replacing, you can get the new tooth colored porcelain ones, so your smile just keeps getting better. Mary sets aside a small amount of money every month towards dental care, and makes all her dentist appointments for the whole year at one time and puts them on her calendar. "I am inspired to do whatever I can to hang on to my original choppers. Flossing, water-picking, brushing, and regular checkups seem a small price to pay for the very sizable benefits of "keeping my original equipment."

Brain Power

Now for some really good news. Scientists used to think that our brains had a finite number of cells; as we aged so did our brains. The picture was grim: lost keys, lost comprehension, memory loss, followed by decline and death.

Old Brains Work Smarter

But thanks to new imaging technology (namely MRI's and functional MRI's) scientists made some startling discoveries. The brain does not have a finite number of brain cells. It can make new ones. Scientists call this "neuroplasticity," the brain can create new cells throughout its entire life, not just the early years. Experience can actually change both the brain's physical structure and functional organization. So while an older brain does slow down when it comes to processing calculations, it does continues to make new connections, and is better than the younger brain at coming to wiser, more meaningful conclusions.

Pathways to Wisdom

A flexible brain has multiple pathways to solve problems. The older executive may not be able to hold *every* bit of information in the forefront of his brain as he did when he was young, but he knows where to look for it when he needs it. Furthermore, the special trick of the older brain is to gather all the information and bring it to a central spot for processing without stopping along the way to consider if the information from that particular collection is applicable. The time taken by younger brains to sort as they go leaves them an even smaller bucket of data from which to draw meaningful conclusions and slows down the process.

An older person can solve problems by calling up a many layered array of possible solutions and then throws out the less relevant ones at the end of the process thereby forming a conclusion that takes in more variables than a younger mind. That is wisdom in action. Finally, the clinical evidence that wisdom really does come with age.

Now there are many, many more "old brains" kicking around the earth than ever before. We are still good for many more years of wisdom. Like old presidents who have risen to the top of their ladders, and then find themselves out of a job, we have a lot to offer the world.

It is time for an evolutionary leap. As with many things we have taken on, the Boomers are about to change the face of aging. Timothy Leary told us back in 1966 to "Mutate, Baby, Mutate!" and it looks like we might do just that! Think about it. Our mature brain's specialty is networking for wisdom. We are in an age where data is so easily found on any computer, we are perfectly poised to help solve some of the world's pressing problems. There may be no stopping us and the generations to come will last longer still. Imagine where we will be, just a few generations forward.

"Take your life in your own hands, and what happens?
A terrible thing: no one to blame."

Erica Jong

CHAPTER ELEVEN
The Aging Plan:
Creating Your Best Future

In which

Mary Boone and Tracey

take their stand for a life well lived.

For joy and vigor, humor and love,

for now and as long

as there is breath (and wine).

Here is the good news: the new "old age" now begins at eighty-five. This is amazing when you consider that just twenty years ago, it was seventy-five. When it comes to aging, the two goals of the more enlightened geriatric doctors are probably the same as yours: independence and contentment. How do you achieve those two marvelous goals? Medical research boils it down to these four things: exercise, eat healthy, prevent falls, and keep mentally active. But as gerontologist Dr. Leo Cooney, explains: "You also need to have self-esteem at eighty-five as much as you need it at fourteen. It's really important to feel good about yourself."

How do you ensure that your "golden years" really will be filled with contentment, that you will feel good about your aging self? It is a bit like making a plan to excel in sport or business. First you choose your goal, and then make a plan to achieve that goal. Illness may happen, yes, and you cannot foresee every malady nor stop the aging process because the body has its own hereditary tendencies, its own karma, and we have all made lifestyle choices that affect our elder years. However, much of what we think of as inevitable may be deflected or deferred by having a powerful goal and a good daily routine that is aligned with achieving that goal.

Think of the vigorous and long-living folks we all know and admire. Betty White at age ninety still holds down a demanding full-time job in a TV show "Hot in Cleveland". About age, she said, "It's not a surprise, we knew it was coming—make the most of it. So you may not be as fast on your feet, and the image in your mirror may be a little disappointing, but if you are still functioning and not in pain, gratitude should be the name of the game." This is a quote from her hilarious and wonderfully readable book If You Ask Me, And of Course You Won't, which she found time to write last year at age eighty-nine.

Jack LaLanne, the first modern fitness guru, was as vigorous and alert as ever when he died at age ninety-six, having worked through his regular two-hour exercise regimen the day before. About exercise, he said: "I do it as a therapy. I do it as something to keep me alive. We all need a little discipline. Exercise is my discipline."

George Burns, beloved comedian, continued to work at his craft, bringing joy to millions right up to his death at age 100. Retaining his light touch through all those years, he said about dying: "I don't believe in dying. It's been done. I'm working on a new exit. Besides, I can't die now—I'm booked."

To ensure a good old age, you need to use all your life experiences, all your wisdom, to plan for it. Most of all, you have to focus on what is important to you and create a future that is filled with more of what you value. However unattainable those desires might seem, defining them is the first step. A book we have found useful for sorting out our highest values from a sea of possibilities is Chris Attwood and Janet Bray Attwood's The Passion Test. The authors tell stories of how a clear focus on what is really important to you makes the achievement of even very lofty goals much easier. The book gives you their useful system for discovering what is at the heart of your own desires for a fulfilling life. On their website-www.thepassiontest.com, you will find a free passion profile and how to enroll in their course that helps you keep focused on your passions.

Tips for longer, healthier lives abound in <u>The Blue Zones</u>, a book by Dan Buttoner. It is a fascinating read about places in the world where people regularly live to be 100. Summarized here are the things that stand out: eating lots of fruit and vegetables, less animal foods; less food altogether; moderate exercise every day; drinking lots of water; having friends and family; sharing your knowledge-- contribute. Tracey's dad has his own philosophy: "Drink water, eat garlic, use Vaseline, exercise." (She says, "I was never quite sure what the Vaseline is for, but it does work for cuts and scrapes!")

Think about how you would like your seventies, eighties, nineties, and centenary to unfold. No one can predict the future, but the smart bet is to make plans now for your long, long future. When we had young children, we knew it was a good idea to buy life insurance; our children would be assured food, clothes, and possibly an education if something happened to us. We appointed guardians. Many of us opened college savings accounts for our kids. Why not look at your old age in the same light? Apply the same protective measure to your old age as you did to your own young children. Your now grown children will surely be grateful that you did.

Finally, all good things come to an end, this book and our lives. Whatever you do, get your after-life paperwork in order. In business we like to say, "plan for the exit right from the start." A good exit strategy gives you a feeling of well-being. It is no surprise that our lives will end someday, as Gail Rubin, (aka The Doyenne of Death,) a certified celebrant and author of the book <u>The Good Goodbye: Funeral Planning For Those Who Don't Plan to Die</u>, knows, having officiated at thousands of send offs. This planning is often put off but important work, as Gail says, "Just as talking about sex won't make you pregnant, talking about funerals won't make you dead—and your family will benefit from the conversation." Gail offers support via email to help you get this important conversation started. On her website, www.agoodgoodbye.com, you can download a free ten page planning form, called "A Good Goodbye"

Essential Check List for a Long and Fruitful Future

- **Insurance:** Get Long-Term Health Insurance, an annuity or check to see if a reverse mortgage of your home will provide enough for your care, should you need help in later years.
  Health insurance-check your health insurance coverage for gaps in prescriptions and hospitalization and consider a medical savings account.

- **Medical Care** - Find a doctor or healthcare provider that you like and one that likes you. Your questions should be answered when asked, your phone calls returned, and you should feel respected as an individual, given choices and not treated like an "old" person who is incapable of thinking anymore.

- **Dental Health** - Make sure your teeth are as great as they can be so they will go the distance with you. Be sure your dentist is up on the latest, greatest technology; if not, change dentists.

- **Exercise** - Make a new diet and exercise plan at the start of every season. You know you aren't going for that brisk walk in the winter if you live in Minnesota!

- **Finance** - Take a good hard look at your financial future and make the changes you need right now so you can have enough money to last you a long, long, happy lifetime. Get creative; living in your camper for a year or two while you pay off debt might be fun!

- **De-clutter** - Get your house in order; make sure it is fixed up safe and tidy. (Don't leave this task to your kids--they will resent it and rightly so!)

- **Legal Paperwork** - Get your legal house in order: living will, will, medical power of attorney, etc., lists of who to call when you die and details of your preferred send off.

- **Engage in Life** - Be sure you have some interests besides your career before you retire. As you age, contemplate how you can become a relevant, useful resource for your world as a member of the "wisdom set."

EPILOGUE:
Walking the Talk

We had finished our book and felt great about that. We were feeling quite virtuous and decided to walk up a local mountain near Mary Boone's house. Then a wonderful thing happened: "We were passed on one of the extra steep bits by what I perceived as an 'old woman.' She was slim, with a gray pony tail and a lot of character in her face. It shocked us to see that she did not seem to be breathing hard at all as she lightly jogged past us, waving as she rounded the bend on her way to the peak."

Some of the self-congratulations for our efforts began to fade as we watched her and it started us talking about forming some new goals. We both said, "I want to be like that 'old' woman, and soon!" Move it or lose it. How many times have you heard or said that and then headed to the refrigerator for a snack because you were ready to start exercising, but later, tomorrow maybe, just not right now?

If you are looking for inspiration to start your fitness program, you don't have to move to New Hampshire, where many older adults routinely climb the 4,000 footers, the collection of forty-eight mountains that soar above our hills and valleys. These old timers clearly know that strength training builds brain power!

Inspired by this "two for one" body/brain deal, Tracey and Mary are working out a schedule of enjoyable daily activities that should keep us feeling and thinking young for the years to come. The new summer season has Mary running again and Tracey has taken up SUP-stand up paddle-boarding!

We suggest you start your weight training program today, and figure out a way to make it fun! Take along friends, or make new ones for mutual inspiration. Think where you might end up with all the new brain cells popping around in your heads!

Today is a beautiful day; the sun is shining and the temperature has risen above freezing at last, so we are off to take brain and body for a nice long hike. We hope to meet you out there on the road!

RESOURCES AND REFERENCES

We gathered the information in this book from many sources in magazines, journals, books, and on various web sites. Some are sited in the text and this list of links and references may be useful to you on your journey into caregiving and aging.

Websites:

www.mdvip.com
www.epill.com
www.caregiverssupportnetwork.org
http://www.cdc.gov/nchs/data/hus/hus10.pdf
http://transgenerational.org/aging/demographics.htm
www.aarp.org
www.aaa.com
http://seniordriving.aaa.com/?zip=10014
www.stopfalls.org
www.uspreventiveservicestaskforce.org
http://www.ncbi.nlm.nih.gov
http://www.eldercareteam.com/public/710.cfm
http://guidetohealthyaging.usseniorcitizen.com/natural-treatment-for-cellulitis
http://www.texasagingnetwork.com/caregivers-corner/cellulitis.htm
http://www.globalaging.org/health/us/2006/dehydration.htm
http://nurs211f07researchfinal.blogspot.com/2007/12/preventing-dehydration-in-elderly.html
http://www.freedrinkingwater.com/water-education/water-senior.htm
http://www.buzzle.com/articles/signs-of-dehydration-in-the-elderly.html
http://www.rnjournal.com/journal_of_nursing/malnutrition_in_the_elderly_an_unrecognized_health_issue.htm
http://seniorservicesinvernessflorida.com/hunger-and-senior-citizens
http://caregivingcompanion.com/senior-citizen-care-combating-elder-malnutrition-home-care-companies-assisted-home-care-at-home-caregivers

http://www.livestrong.com/article/510035-how-to-prevent-and-treat-malnutrition

http://www.cdc.gov/heartdisease/statistics.htm

The report includes: Facts, Maps and Statistics, Statistical Reports, Morbidity and Mortality Weekly Reports (MMWRs)

http://www.theheartfoundation.org/heart-disease-facts/heart-disease-statistics

Provides information about heart disease; statistics, how to reduce heart disease, and additional links to other resources

www.buzzle.com

www.globalaging.org

www.nihseniorhealth.gov National Institute Of Health

http://www.nia.nih.gov National Institute On Aging

http://www.knowyourteeth.com Academy of General Dentistry

http://www.nlm.nih.gov/medlineplus/anesthesia.html

http://www.mayoclinic.com/health/aging-parents/HA00082

www.costo.com

www.seniorsuperstores.com

www.activeforever.com

www.eldergym.com

www.strongerseniors.com

www.kintzltc.com

www.ltcfeds.com

http://publications.usa.gov/USAPubs.php?PubID=5879 Long Term Care Insurance info

www.centerpointe.com

www.best-personal-growth-resources.com/easy-meditation.html

www.siddhayogabookstore.org/meditationinstructions.aspx

link to a book and CD set for learning meditation

http://www.alert-1.com/do-you-need-medical-alert-quiz/do-i-need-quiz.aspx

www.alert-1.com

www.aoa.gov Administration on Aging, a department of the US Department of Health and Human Services

www.cdc.gov Center for Disease Control

www.cms.gov Medicare and Medicaid info

www.ssa.gov Social Security Administration

www.naela.org National Academy of Elder Law Attorneys, Inc.

http://www.rosalynncarter.org Rosalyn Carter Institute For Caregiving

http://www.biomedcentral.com/1471-2474/12/105 article on hip fracture

http://www.ncbi.nlm.nih.gov/pmc/articles/PMC2552979/ Anesthesia article